Caring for
an Aging Parent

D1233958

Golden Age Books
Perspectives on Aging

Caring for an Aging Parent

Have I Done All I Can?

Avis Jane Ball

PROMETHEUS BOOKS

Buffalo, New York

The publisher gratefully acknowledges *The Wall Street Journal* for permission to reprint paragraphs appearing on pages 123 and 133 of this volume. Copyright by Dow Jones & Company, Inc. 1979. All Rights Reserved.

Published 1986 by Prometheus Books
700 East Amherst Street, Buffalo, New York 14215

Library of Congress Cataloging-in-Publication Data

Ball, Avis Jane, 1912-
    Caring for an aging parent.
    (Golden Age Books)
    Rev. ed. of: What shall I do with a hundred years?
c1982.
    1. Parents, Aged—Care and hygiene—United States.
2. Parents, Aged—United States—Family relationships.
3. Adult children—United States—Family relationships.
4. Parent and child—United States. I. Ball, Avis Jane,
1912-   What shall I do with a hundred years?
II. Title.
HQ1064.U5B24 1986   306.8'7   86-18664
ISBN 0-87975-368-4
ISBN 0-87975-364-1 (pbk.)

Printed in the United States of America

Foreword

Each year thousands of persons in the United States face the struggles and the moral decisions that Avis Jane Ball faced in taking care of her aging father. With our increased life expectancy, more and more people are encountering the difficulties of seeing their parents become old, infirm, senile, and totally dependent. Perhaps no dilemma is more difficult than that which is felt by loving children who see their once strong, intelligent, articulate, productive parents become mean, obstinate, cantankerous, and infirm. It is not easy to know what to do when those you love want to remain in familiar surroundings of their own homes and virtually demand 24-hour-a-day attention and nursing care. This ministry of love can become a virtual sentence to slavery.

Caring for an Aging Parent is the story of one person's pilgrimage in facing the issues out of a background of responsibility, love, and faith. Avis Jane Ball has agonized through all the emotions of loss, fear, anger, and resentment, and has lived in that faint valley of hope, trying to make things work out for her father. She was not able to do everything that she wanted to do. She finally decided to do what she had to do. Her experiences can serve well to lighten the load for all of us as we read her poignant account. I have been privileged to know the author as she formulated her thoughts, created her manuscript, and sought her publisher in order to tell for others' benefit how lonely those decisions and actions are. This book will serve as an effective tool for ministers, priests and rabbis, for those who work in institutions taking care of the aged, for neighbors who see the changes that time brings, and especially for the "lonely ones" who take care of their aged and infirm parents.

Donald H. Welsh
United Methodist Clergyman
Chief of Chaplain Service,
Virginia Medical Center
Fresno, California

Donald H. Welsh has conducted a regular weekly educational program "Coping With Loss." During the last eight years several thousand persons have attended the class from such diverse backgrounds as hospital inpatients and outpatients, nursing students from local colleges and universities, psychology graduate students, hospital staff members, widows, divorced persons, biblical seminary students, local pastors and persons experiencing various forms of grief. He is a frequent lecturer throughout central California where he conducts seminars and workshops on the topics "Understanding Human Grief" and "Death and Dying."

I dedicate this book

To my husband
     who was generous
     with his support
     and
To my father
     who was a fine man
     and
To those Lonely Ones.

Prologue

The freeway ribboned ahead, lonely, deserted, on a dismal fall afternoon, with little traffic to interrupt my thinking. The landscape spun by, trees stark and bare, their once brilliant leaves, now brown and brittle, scattering along the pavement. The atmosphere was mood-matching after closing the cottage with a sunken feeling that I had deserted the tiny retreat.

Speeding toward home, I was pursued by the memory of another happier occasion, five years before. On a sweltering July morning, my daughter and I had made that same two-hundred-mile drive to welcome my father, recently retired at age eighty-five from a job in the Midwest. Despite his reluctance to stop working, we had persuaded him to move east to his boyhood town to an apartment three blocks from our home, within walking distance of stores and the library. We had painted the rooms, made new draperies, put fresh linen on the bed, and had hung a picture of a crimson geranium, once treasured in my parents' home. Driving homeward, then, I visualized the appreciative smile of the tall, strong, outgoing, extraordinary man. My father!

The exhilaration of the past was lost now in a sense of foreboding that accelerated with the passing of each mile. An abrupt change had taken place in my father. Still physically strong, he walked with the stride that had been his trademark throughout

9

the years. But a cataract on each eye, for which he refused surgery, made him dependent upon a white cane, deprived him of the companionship of books and the daily paper, and prevented his work on a manuscript for a book of his own. Now, with the deterioration of his mind, he was confused, neglected personal cleanliness, and could care less whether or not I cleaned his rooms. The man with the mind of a genius—the loving, considerate parent—had become childish, petulant, frantic, arbitrary! (I avoided the words *senile* and *incompetent*.) And I, who from childhood had been near and dear to my father, was having to cope with his idiosyncrasies and with idiosyncrasies of my own, growing from his, like the snake-covered head of an ugly Medusa.

It was beginning to rain. I sought inner strength. Trying to assure myself that I cared about my father enough to give his needs priority over mine, I cried aloud, "Oh, how lonely!" and flipped the windshield wiper into action as if to dry my tears. Remembering my father's infantile behavior of recent months, I exploded, "Oh, how childish!" I pressed the accelerator to the speed limit and wound up the window, for fear a passing motorist might overhear. I was ashamed and frustrated; and angry that I, in good health, dreaded facing my father's frailty. Were others in a like situation as frustrated as I? Did they ever complain? Were they annoyed or resentful sometimes toward the one in their charge, toward themselves for becoming resentful? Did they, too, feel as if they were fighting for their lives, as if trapped into choosing between their own lives and the life of the person who was disabled? Was anyone else, with a problem similar to mine, overwhelmed by a cauldron of mixed emotions: love, despair, compassion, guilt, utter loss? I wondered. I was sixty-two years old, and the fact that I was approaching life as a senior citizen colored my thinking, for the care of my father made me feel as if I had been forced to live old age twice.

When I was younger, how often had I heard people remark, "Now that I'm retired and have fewer responsibilities, I can relax and enjoy life." Seldom have I heard this said in recent years, for the situation has been changing with the dramatic escalation of longevity. The preliminary unpublished 1980 census figures from the Bureau of Census Office in Washington, D.C., show that (in round figures) 32,000 people in the United States were one hundred years of age or older, and 46,000 people were ninety-five years of age. One might suspect that many people in their seventies and even eighties, with retirement traumas of their own, will have to assume the care of parents or relatives of an older generation, or at the very least, be forced to make decisions in their behalf. Year by year, while longevity was escalating, my own life was being affected, as I took care of my father.

The November 10, 1980 issue of the *San Francisco Chronicle* carried an article from the New York News Syndicate with a revealing statement:

> Some psychologists say that the responsibility of caring for aging parents is becoming the major family problem—outstripping marital problems, childrearing, personal identity crisis, finances.

"No one can comprehend the trauma of such an experience," says a friend, "until he has had the day-to-day responsibility of an older disabled person." I concur, for heretofore I myself had never understood. Even so, at the time of my own involvement in the care of my father, I was not certain that the experience completed my understanding of the loyalty I owed to him, to my husband, to our two daughters, and to myself!

The experiences in this account will, I hope, enlighten those who have never watched at firsthand the slow death caused by deteriorating mental health of an aged person; help them refrain from being judgmental; and encourage them to support friends and relatives who, day after day and with little respite, cope with the mental, physical, and emotional incapacities and insecurities of someone who is older.

The chapters that follow contain a real-life exposé for those who study gerontology, grief, and death and dying, to better

Chapter One

Expectancy was the word of the day. The upturned faces of a cluster of people watched the plane as it circled over the airfield. Amy, our ten-year-old, leaning backward to scan the sky, almost keeled over with glee as she called out, "Grandfather waved from a window." Janice, fourteen, insisted, "I saw him reach for is briefcase." This was always the game on his annual fall visit: who would be the first to catch sight of Grandfather Yale?

The fence with its sign, NO VISITORS ALLOWED, controlled our impatience. People chattered excitedly: "There it is— the flight from Detroit—right on time," while we kept assuring each other. "Here he comes. Oh, here he comes."

In that moment, we were bursting with excitement as we watched the plane's "hatch" spring open like an enormous cargo of treasure and the steps reach down, down from the plane to the ground. The stewardess in the doorway called to the passengers, "Have a good day," with no idea of how good the day was for the Ball family. The thought that a week later we would be weeping "good-bye" was buried deep in our hearts. Today we had TODAY. A good day, indeed.

Behind the stewardess appeared a tall, distinguished-looking gentleman who acknowledged his farewell with a nod. At the foot of the steps, he turned to shake hands with another man. I laughed. Unless Dad had started a conversation with his seatmate, the flight would have been boring.

Nearby, an amateur band began to blare, as a delegation with a welcome sign surrounded a young couple just arriving.

"It's a salute to you, too," I bantered in my father's embrace. "Welcome home. Oh, welcome home."

"Honey Jane," he said—my pet name since childhood— "where's John?"

"Daddy had to make deliveries for the store," Amy said.

Her grandfather leaned toward her and Amy giggled and threw herself into his arms. He kissed Janice who shyly snuggled her hand into his. In the excitement, he knocked over his brief-case. He chuckled apologetically. "Would you believe it? I've mislaid my traveller's checks."

Not even this calamity could spoil the occasion, for my fa-ther's arrival was as exciting as Christmas. To the children, who for weeks had been making plans for his visit, Grandfather Yale was an example of a perfect grandparent. He made sport of Amy and Jan showering him with rice, exclaimed over the lyrics of their favorite recordings, applauded their amateur dance recitals, and proudly became a card-carrying honorary member of their neighborhood club. He charmed them with true stories about the time he was best man in the "Opera House" for the wedding of two midgets from the Barnum Circus; about working in his fa-ther's grocery where farmers embarrassed him as a teenager with, "My, how you do grow"; about a racer in our town's past who, when he yelled "whoa," trained his horse to run; and about the little girl he loved as a child, later to become their grandmother.

Always, Dad's coming placed me in a controversial position, with the girls who bemoaned "wasting" time in school during his visit and complained that I monopolized him, and with John who could not understand why Dad and I stayed up late to talk, or how I had the temerity to tease and boss my father.

"It's disrespectful," insisted John, who had never enjoyed such rapport with his own father.

Dad laughed. "You're right. Honey Jane doesn't respect my dignity." A private joke between us for years.

Over warm milk toast and cheddar cheese, I shared the day-to-day problems of rearing the girls. I complained, "In the past, parents depended upon children to follow their upbringing; but now there are too many pressures outside the home."

My father was reassuring. "When your mother and I raised you and your brother Frank, my mother used to insist, 'You have to keep repeating rules until children get the point.'" He scratched his head thoughtfully. "It seems to me young people have a right to make their own mistakes and to learn from them; these days, they're more advanced than we were at their age, but we under-rate their intelligence. I have confidence in today's youth." He reached across the table to press my hand. "Especially your two girls and Frank's three children. How your mother would have enjoyed them."

Moments like these strengthened between us a bond of long-ing for my mother. I began to reminisce. "Remember how Mom used to say that any woman could have you if she could get you?"

Dad chuckled and recalled her return, in later years, to our small-town church, where she told the preacher, "On this very spot a boy kissed a girl."

The reverend looked shocked. "You don't mean in this holy place?"

Mother looked him in the eye and asked, "Would you have preferred that Tom kissed me in the American Legion Hall?"

There were other memories of Mother. I said, "When she divided groceries from our cupboard with a needy family, I never heard you criticize her."

Dad looked astonished, "But I was proud of her."

Even when Dad travelled on business, he and Mother shared an unusual closeness. She packed tiny marigolds in wet cotton, one to wear each day in his buttonhole, and tucked "train letters" from us all into his suitcase.

"She was a gallant lady." My father began to relive the days in Detroit when at fifty-seven he became unemployed, when repeatedly he was told, "Sorry, you're too old." He said, "I'll never forget how hard it was for your mother, and for you children, too."

After my mother's death, those of us who had been included in the love that she and my father shared watched helplessly as Dad divided between us the accumulated treasures of their married life, as he moved to a cell-like room in a men's hotel, and then moved again to a shabby efficiency apartment in the suburbs.

Once an editor and executive director of sales, my father became a salesman in a men's clothing store, then a desk attendant in a social club, and was now a clerk in a credit office; after hours, he worked on a book about discrimination against the aged—its title, "A Search for Understanding."

He said, "I owe it to your mother to finish my book—to change conditions if only for a few." He began to pace the floor, as he relived the trauma of his unemployment.

Unable to endure watching him suffer, I attempted to shift the subject. "Since you began working at the credit office, how much time have you missed?"

He sat down again, thought for a moment, and said, "In ten years, I've taken only four days' sick leave."

The experience of extended unemployment had left a mark on my father; the hurts were deep-seated, increasing his feeling of insecurity. Few who knew him suspected that the man who listened to their problems with such empathy lacked self-confidence. Mornings, while he was shaving, his desperation exploded. As I lay in bed, burying my head in the pillow, I hoped John and the children would not hear Dad's cursing, so foreign to his gentle nature.

But nothing could dampen spirits at our annual celebration in an elite restaurant as my father's guests. John took me aside and protested Dad spending the money. I reminded John that this compensated my father for the time when he had to borrow from us. Hosting the dinner was crucial to Dad's sense of personal worth.

At home, afterward, Jan and Amy pleaded with their grandfather to extend his stay. They beat pots and pans with kitchen spoons, paraded with their toy Manchester—hanging from his neck a placard that begged, PLEASE STAY. Engrossed in their play picketing, they were unaware of the tears in their grandfather's eyes.

The next morning, at the airport, we watched the plane lift into the sky, gradually dwindling until it looked like a bird heading for the clouds—the only tangible evidence of an experience that now seemed a dream.

Returning to the car, Jan burst into tears. Solemnly, Amy distributed paper handkerchiefs to Jan and me, and said, "I can't wait. I just can't wait until next year—when Grandfather comes again."

Chapter Two

"Retirement's not all it's cracked up to be," wrote my father. Still employed at age eighty-five, he was haunted by a picture he had seen of some elderly men seated on a park bench. Beneath the picture a caption read: "Too old to work, too young to die." He recalled a retiree who was presented with a watch at a testimonial dinner and, upon returning to visit the office, was ignored by employees who were preoccupied with their work. He never forgot how his father, after retirement, filled in time in the park with other older men who had nothing to do.

My letters kept urging Dad to consider retiring close to us.

"But a man needs a daily schedule to keep from going down-hill," he protested. "Your mother and I always agreed we'd never become a burden to you children."

From my own viewpoint, there were other considerations. Even though by this time the girls were adults, I could not leave home for an extended period of time. Supposing Dad became ill—too far away for me to take care of him? Or supposing he were to die—alone?

Between the lines of my father's letters, I began to detect a wistfulness for the town where he and my mother had been raised. I persisted, "You could devote more time to your book and catch up on your reading; then, of course, in the summer you'd visit us at the cottage."

"Summer home," he corrected. "I've told people at the office you've invited me to visit your summer home."

One evening when I answered the phone, the clatter of coins alerted me to a long distance call from a public booth. Dad's voice was husky. "If I retired, how could I move all my belongings? Especially my research materials?"

"That's no problem," I said. "John insists he'll come for you—bag and baggage."

"But it's a seven-hundred-mile drive."

"Frank can't leave Ohio, so John insists." I pressed for an immediate decision: "Get out your suitcase and start packing. That's an order!"

"You're bossing me, young lady." Dad's laughter, mixed with tears, came over the wire. "It's a big step." There was silence for a moment, then suddenly he said, "All right. I'll come."

We sprang into action. After enlisting the help of friends to truck furniture from our house to a nearby apartment, John left for the Midwest to get Dad, while Amy (home from college) helped me clean and paint. Jan, now married to a Navy man, lived in the far west.

The apartment vibrated with excitement as we welcomed my father. Home at last!

"You've performed a miracle," he said, as he ran his fingers over the blue wallpaper above the counter in the kitchenette; opened the refrigerator; and stepped to the picture window to look onto the lawn. Dad stood thoughtfully in front of the geranium print, his and my mother's favorite.

I asked, "Did I write that this building was once a hospital, and your living room the surgery?"

He laughed. "I'll invite friends to visit me in surgery."

I was hesitant. "When do you think you'll feel able to leave for the cottage?"

"You mean summer home," he corrected. "Tomorrow, of course, bright and early."

The next morning, as we headed for The Haven, my father appeared refreshed. If this was a sample of aging, there was little to dread, for even after we reached the cottage, he showed no sign of weariness. He insisted on contributing toward groceries; and when I protested, he argued, "If I rented a place in this resort area, it would cost a fortune."

There were adjustments for all of us. For Dad, there was lack of privacy in a room with only a curtain between John's and mine. For me and John, there was the squeaking of bedsprings as Dad tossed and turned, sometimes cursing in his sleep. For Amy, who had a "thing" about pollution, her grandfather's cigar stubs littering the yard.

My father's hobbies were taking long walks, reading mysteries or more serious books by Rollo May and Victor Frankl, and playing solitaire or a game of Scrabble. Sometimes he wandered to the settlement's shuffleboard court in search of companionship. Sometimes I invited professional men to meet my father for coffee, but they never came. Sometimes, wistfully, Dad shared portions of letters from Rex Winters, a friend from credit bureau days who reported that the office was retiring employees at sixty-five. I was comforted by the thought that Dad had decided to leave before the bureau had insisted, "You're through."

Those were solitary days for one who had been in the mainstream of life; but revelling in the beauty around The Haven, Dad never complained. More than once, he exclaimed, "Just look at the different shades of green in the forest! Of the four hundred cottages, yours has the loveliest setting."

The summer was enriched by letters from Jan whose experiences as an art teacher delighted my father. He said, "The school will have to go a long ways to find a teacher as creative as Jan."

The summer was spiced with controversial discussions between Amy and her grandfather, about her college life, her fiance, her work at a nearby store, and about psychology and religion. Dad chuckled over her unconventional viewpoints, and said of her fiance, "He'll have to be a good man to deserve our Amy."

As autumn began to tint the forest, we boxed up the cottage for the winter. Returning to town, Dad went at once to the bank, opened a checking account, and rented a safe deposit box jointly in his name and mine. "In case of an emergecy," he explained, "I'm not getting any younger." I shrugged off the emergency, for my father seemed ageless. He visited the local employment bureau to apply for part-time work—a strange sight, the white-haired gentleman standing in line with applicants who were years younger.

When no job materialized, my father settled down during the daytime to write his book, while at night he attended meetings of the city council and the local school board to keep abreast of community affairs. On index cards stored in his pocket, he filed names of townspeople, including supermarket employees, with whom he lingered to visit.

The local newspaper interviewed the eighty-five-year-old gentleman who had not retired from life, and published a feature entitled "He's Too Busy at 85, Remembering, But Looking Ahead." My father was quoted:

WE MUST MAINTAIN PERSONAL INTEGRITY

The kids are taking an interest in problems as a matter of principle. I feel that peaceful demonstrations are an American right. If a man can't disagree with me, then I'm afraid to test my own convictions. I cannot avoid the conviction that so many have uttered that we adults have not measured up to our own idealism.

His personal interests, the paper reported, were educational reform, problems of the aged, vocational education, and school taxes. "The biggest problem for society to face," he said, "was just that: bigness. Decision making is being moved farther away from the people."

Proud of the newspaper photo that captured Dad's strength of character, and the article that capsuled his sense of purpose and the integrity he championed, I sent copies to old friends, and of course one to my brother. His friends wrote their congratulations, and Frank responded in a poignant letter expressing his love and admiration.

Businessmen invited Dad to join them for coffee daily in the local restaurant. He began to challenge their apathy toward local and world events. He pricked the conscience of the school board when it threatened to dismiss a coach whose hair was long. In a letter to the paper, he poked fun at the fact that his own ancestors' hair was long, too. People began to ask if he planned to run for City Council. The Kiwanis Club invited him to lecture and honored him with a standing ovation.

A young businessman, Henry Clark, invited Dad to a Saturday breakfast where every week men from varied occupations and religious faiths discussed their convictions. Their search for happiness and peace of mind frustrated my father, for he had never stopped caring since his speech in college that ended with, "Yours for a better world here and now." He asked the men how they could attain peace while poverty was rampant throughout the world. They spoke ardently of faith. Dad said he had lost his when he became unemployed, and exploded over the injustice of age discrimination. They said they loved him. Deeply touched, Dad told me, "They keep inviting me to return in spite of our positions at opposite poles." He affectionately called the group his "Club."

The tall man with white hair, who in winter never wore a hat or rubbers, became a figurehead in town. Townspeople were intrigued with the elder citizen who was advanced in his thinking, concerned about community needs, and interested in their opinions. They became accustomed to his habitually offered advice: "Learn one thing everyday," then jokingly, "but not more than one." Whenever they greeted him with "How are you today, Mr. Yale?" they learned to respect his answer, "Oh, normally abnormal."

Chapter Three

"If I increase your father's rent, will it be a hardship for him?" The landlady's question startled me; her brittle tone of voice belied her concern.

My answer was abrupt. "You'll have to ask *him*." Even if I had known the amount of my father's income, I would have been unwilling to act as his spokesman.

Mrs. Bennett's eyes were piercing. "Property taxes have increased. So has the water bill. I may be forced to increase the rent. . . ."

I interrupted, "Why don't you discuss it with my father?"

An undercurrent of hostility prepared me for her blunt reply. "Last week when the plumber came, the bathroom was filthy. You father must keep the place clean."

"Tell that to him." I bit my tongue, unable to adjust to the role of parent to my father.

Dad was a reliable tenant who paid his rent on time. He was courteous and cooperatrive, offering in winter to share the cost of snow removal. (He even suggested shoveling the snow himself, heaven forbid!) It was clear, however, that Mrs. Bennett held me responsible for keeping his apartment clean.

The next day, when I appeared at Dad's door, armed with dustpan, pail, and rags, he was apologetic about my doing the cleaning. A week later, he said it would be inconvenient to move his writing materials out of my way. The third week, before I arrived, he scrubbed the linoleum with cleansing powder, removing the wax I had applied.

On hands and knees, I scrubbed the floor again, applied a fresh coat of wax, and turned a deaf ear to Dad's protests of "Why bother?" From then on, "Why bother?" became a barricade between us: "Why bother?" when I suggested he take a walk while I worked, "Why bother?" when I teased that no man could clean as well as a woman. In desperation, I phoned Frank, who urged me not to get excited. Overwhelmed by a battle that seemed hopeless, I felt utterly alone.

As each week began, I dreaded arguing with my father about cleaning. I sneaked into his apartment when he went to the barber shop or the public library. I degreased the stove and scoured the bathroom sink and tub, with my stomach turning a tailspin. I cleaned the oily hair and scalp crud from Dad's comb. On my knees, I wiped up the urine stain beneath the toilet and prayed the plumber would not be summoned again. Sometimes, when a confrontation with my father seemed inevitable, and the accumulating soil made the task intolerable, I procrastinated, feeling like a parent neglecting to discipline a child.

Other times the problems were pushed aside by special events, such as a shower for Dad on Jan's return for a visit, with gifts from us all for his apartment. He had never had a shower, Dad told us shyly, as he opened the gaily decorated packages, examined the flowered sheets and pillowcases, and a bathmat with the words, "Keep Klean." Sometimes we had lunch at the cafeteria of a nearby school, where my father rubbed elbows with students and exchanged viewpoints on current issues. Sometimes he visited a boyhood friend, Judge Wilkins, whose photos of old-timers revived memories of the old days.

A traumatic interruption was Amy's broken engagement when Dad phoned daily to ask, "What do you hear from Amy?" Whenever I was depressed, he reassured me. "I have a lot of faith in our Amy. She'll come through."

One day, as I knocked on Dad's door, the shuffling of his house slippers was drowned by the noon whistle. Standing in the doorway, he looked forlorn: his shirt open at the neck, sleeves rolled above the elbow, his lips moving soundlessly as the whistle continued to blast.

The racket ended. Breathing heavily, Dad said that after awakening he had walked in his stocking feet to the refrigerator and opened it to remove a carton of milk. The phone rang, and when he answered, he was startled by his landlady's threat that unless he was quiet she would summon the police.

"Could your typing have awakened her?" I asked, wondering if Mrs. Bennett might have overheard his cursing.

"I haven't used my typewriter today," Dad said. "Besides, the tenants next door assured me they seldom noticed the sound."

When the plumber was called back by the landlady, Dad was skating on thin ice, and taking me with him. In a panic, I considered writing Frank, but recalling his previous philosophical response, thought better of it. Whenever I was tempted to postpone the cleaning, I prayed for a miracle as if the sky might open to reveal angels with mops, pails, and dustcloths. I wondered how I could face Dad with the truth that he had a responsibility to protect Mrs. Bennett's property and to uphold my reputation, since I had secured the apartment for him.

Again, the noon whistle was a forecast of doom. I called through the half-open door. Dad's face was ashen, his hand shaking as he held out a folded paper. The whistle stopped. The paper crackled in the silence as I opened a legal document bordered with his thumb prints. An eviction notice!

Sinking into a chair, I waited for an explanation. Confusion clouded his deep-set eyes and trembled on his lips. "She insisted the apartment was dirty; it really doesn't look bad." He waved a cloth, flipping dust from the table. "She can't be serious about evicting me." He lifted a vase from the bookcase and rubbed the wood vigorously as if this might give him a reprieve.

I promised to do what I could. Blaming myself for not facing the problem head-on long before, I clung to the fading hope that Mrs. Bennett might change her mind.

That afternoon I sought legal counsel. The lawyer's face was sober. "You'd better find your father another rental soon," he said. "Unless you do, the landlady has informed me, she'll take your father to court."

Chapter Four

"Your mother and I always agreed we'd never move in with you or Frank." As if I disputed this, Dad repeated, "We always said we'd never live with our children."

Unable to think of an answer, I remained silent, while he paced back and forth, his shoes pounding the floor. "There's no solution to my problem. No solution at all." The depressing lines that sketched my father's cheeks were taut with despair, his white hair streaked with yellow—an indication, my mother used to say, of emotional stress.

I tried to think of a way to change the subject. Stalling for time, I glanced about the sun-filled room decorated by Amy and me only a year before. The eviction had become a nightmare.

"Of course there's Jan's room at our house," I volunteered.

"No. No!" Dad's chin protruded stubbornly. "I'll never live with you and John. Never!"

Inwardly, I had to admit that sharing our home with my father, on a full-time basis, could prove a strain on us all. It was painful to contemplate that the old days, once so bright, were now in the shadows.

Oh, how I needed Frank! But I decided not to call him, to spare him the worry about Dad's eviction.

Every night, I telephoned my father, schooling my voice to

sound optimistic. Weary of his insistence that I would never find another rental, I said, "I'm as stubborn as you, Dad. I'll find a place. You can depend upon it."

Before long it became clear that neither of us could depend upon it. Where was there another apartment small enough, close to us, and within walking distance of the business district, at a cost within my father's income?

The fragrance of burning fall leaves filled the air; frost chilled me to the bone. Classified ads became of greater importance than the headlines or the weather report. To protect Dad's state of mind, I screened the vacancies by myself, but as I pursued my daily search, he kept appearing—a lonely figure, his shoulders sagging, his face grey with anxiety—searching, too.

Day after day, we examined one vacancy after another, each with its own unique drawbacks: A mammoth old house, re-modelled into apartments where the tenant pointed out a leaky bathtub and the fire hazard of endless extension cords. Another rental, up an open stairway that would be iced-over in winter. Twenty steps to another, where I gasped for breath, while Dad insisted he could manage the steep clim. I begged him to accept a first floor studio, near friendly neighbors, but he exploded, "It's too small and confining. Stop pressuring me." I longed for bed-time and escape into sleep; I felt guilty because I had a permanent home with John to keep me company.

Day and night, desperation haunted me, forcing me to seek help at church gatherings, at the supermarket, at the laundromat—whenever and wherever anyone would listen: "My father needs an apartment. His landlady wants the one he's occupying—for a relative."

One morning, as I searched the classifieds halfheartedly, I found a new ad, and on dialing the phone number, I discovered that three doors from us, the Martin family had a vacancy in their apartment house.

As Dad and I approached the building, I suggested, "Why don't you explain to Mrs. Martin that I'll be cleaning for you regularly?"

He was visibly offended. "Why tell her that? When I pay the rent, the apartment becomes mine to use as I please."

I was desperate. "But Dad, when I've visited you, I've dreaded using your bathroom—it's so dirty."

For a moment I thought he was going to stomp off and leave me, but his hands grasped my shoulders; he stormed, "You can't talk to me that way. You can't."

Unaccustomed to his loss of control, I tried to placate him as we neared the house.

At her back door, Mrs. Martin offered the key and said, "You'd probably like to inspect the apartment by yourselves."

"Nice draperies," commented Dad, as I opened the door. The huge flowers were ugly and faded, the hems hung loose, reminding me of a woman in a sloppy dress. But the room was cheerful, with a dinette at one end, then a kitchenette, and next to the bedroom a small bath.

Dad pointed to a corner of the living room. "We could put my easy chair there, and the television against the opposite wall. I could work on my book in the dinette." He hesitated. "But you said the rent is an increase of fifteen dollars."

I controlled an impulse to scream. "But you have no choice, Dad. There are no other vacancies."

He opened a cupboard in the kitchen and closed it, wandered through the bedroom to the bathroom, and pushed aside the shower curtain. He restlessly paced back and forth into the kitchen again, peering into the cupboard and the small, old-fashioned refrigerator.

"Mrs. Martin will be wondering about us," I said. "We've been here for over a half hour."

He hesitated at the kitchen door. "I just don't know. I just don't know about the extra rent. . . ."

"It's worth it, Dad. There's so much more space."

"If I can manage the added expense. . . ." he mused.

I tried to be jocular. "You could give up smoking, to save. . . ."

His face turned white with anger.

Longing for my brother's support, I said, "Frank would urge you to take it. I know he would."

Dad sighed. "I suppose you're right."

Before he could change his mind, I hurried toward the door. He followed. My relief was shattered by the realization that the eviction had robbed me of a father who had been self-reliant. The man who had lived independently, with courage and dignity, seemed no longer able to manage on his own. I had never expected to have the responsibility of making decisions for another adult. For the first time in my life, I faced a problem I could not share with my father.

Chapter Five

"I just can't leave," Dad said, the night before moving day. I was sure I had misunderstood, but he repeated, "I can't leave this apartment."

After a week of turmoil, when Dad had turned down a friend's offer of a truck, forcing me to search for a mover, I was in no mood to deal with his objections. I said, "You have no choice. Your landlady won't allow you to stay here. I'm sure, once you're settled in the new place, you'll enjoy it."

He shook his head and ran his fingers nervously through his hair. Surrounding the easy chair where he was sitting were boxes he had packed, a visible contradiction to his determination not to move.

The following morning, I phoned my father to remind him that the movers were due at four, found that his night's rest had not altered his state of mind, and visualized him shaking his head as he insisted again, "I just don't know what to do. I don't see how I can leave."

Shortly before the movers were due, I went to the apartment building, discovering a freshly-shoveled path in the snow leading to the door. My father was in his easy chair. His skin was ashen, his lips purple; he said, "I shoveled a path for the movers."

I gasped. "You didn't! Not at your age."

He was stubborn, his independence struggling to survive. "It didn't hurt me. Not a bit." He was breathing heavily.

When the movers arrived, I whispered to the driver that I feared my father might collapse.

"Don't worry, Ma'am," he said. "I know how to take care of old people. I'm on the first aid squad."

While the men loaded the truck, I took advantage of my father's confusion and led him, unresisting, to the car. At his new home, I helped him through the snowpath to the door.

Fretting like a child, he asked, "Have I done the right thing? Should I have stayed in the other place?"

I ignored his questions, and as we entered the apartment, I suggested that he turn up the thermostat. "It does seem more comfortable here," he admitted.

Tracking snow, the men brought in boxes of books, trying to avoid Dad in the center of the room. They assembled the bed and unloaded the dresser, the dinette table, a floor lamp, and box after box of personal belongings. Wherever they moved, my father stood in their path, until they placed his easy chair in the corner. With a sigh, he sat down, and with shaking hands he wrote a check and gave it to the driver.

The door slammed. Dad asked, "Is there anything to eat?"

"Can't you smell the pot roast?" I asked. "John will be here soon to help celebrate your new home."

Dad ate heartily, and his eyes began to lose their desperation. He said, "It does seem like home, now that my pictures are on the wall and the furniture is in place."

Later, I phoned the doctor and described Dad's reluctance to move, his shovelling the snow, his ashen complexion and purple lips.

"Changing to unfamiliar surroundings often makes older people feel uprooted," the doctor said. "His confusion is from hardening of the arteries. He'll feel better after a good night's rest."

The doctor was right. The next morning, the problems of

moving seemed to have evaporated. Dad arose early; took a cold shower; prepared coffee, toast, and a boiled egg; then returned with me to his former residence to see that nothing had been overlooked.

Mrs. Bennett's heels clicked on the bare floor as she approached the door.

I asked, "What about a refund of my father's downpayment?"

Her answer was crisp. "We'll see—after I've cleaned the place."

I was firm. "No. I'll clean it myself."

She stood with her hands on her hips. "You'll have to wash the walls."

Tempted to remind her that I had painted the walls, I held my tongue, watched with relief as she left, then faced another battle with Dad, who begged me to let him help. In no mood to have him underfoot, I told him it was hard to work around a man's feet, and breathed a sigh of relief as he left reluctantly.

Determined to force the landlady to make a refund, I washed and rinsed the walls, dusted the built-in bookcases, scrubbed the hard-water ring in the bathtub, turned on the vacuum, and sang to the top of my lungs, mischievously hoping the noise would send a message through the open register to the landlady's quarters.

John phoned to ask about dinner. I blew up, told him the day had been a disaster, and that he'd have to fend for himself.

At nine that evening, I returned to my father and announced, "The job's finished. Your lease in the other apartment ends at midnight. I suggest you prepare a statement for the landlady to sign, stating that she's satisfied with the condition of the rooms; otherwise, she may blame you for any damage done by new tenants."

When we knocked on her door, the landlady looked surprised. She followed us to the apartment; inspected it, room by room; signed the statement Dad handed her; and wrote a check for the deposit. Like two conniving children, Dad and I grinned at each other.

A chapter was ending, as I pulled the outer door shut and said, "She never noticed the dust I left on the air conditioner."

"Trust you," chuckled Dad.

Under the street light, I grinned at him. "I left Mrs. Bennett a gift in the service cellar."

Dad was curious. "What was it?"

I laughed. "I left your mop pail. It leaks!"

Chapter Six

I waved to the postman from the porch. There was no mail, but thumbtacked to the door was a slip of paper with a message in my father's meticulous script:

> I'm leaving town.
> Have a good trip to the cottage,
> And have a good life!
>
> Love, Dad

Whenever we left for The Haven, it was typical of my father to wish us well, but his "have a good life" seemed like a veiled threat, an indication of deepening depression—an added problem to his deteriorating eyesight, for which he refused surgery.

Loading supplies into the car, John called, "With Monday off, we'll have a good long weekend."

"Have a good life." The words' double meaning drove me to call Frank, who by this time had learned that Dad had moved.

As usual, Frank was philosophical. "I phoned Dad last night; he said he's enjoying his new home and that you've accomplished another miracle."

I repeated the last sentence of Dad's note: "Have a good life," adding, "It's not the first time he's threatened to leave town. He's even purchased an overnight bag."

"He has a right to leave if he chooses," Frank said.

I asked, "But what shall I do if the police phone me from another town to come and get him?"

"We'll face that when it happens," Frank said.

His easy attitude was beginning to irritate me, because the miles separated him from the problems that I was having to face close at hand.

I was torn between taking Dad to The Haven or leaving him on his own. Then I decided that the cottage was too cool and damp. Besides, John needed a vacation from the problem, and this time his needs should take precedence over my father's. I slammed the door on the decision and hurried to the car where John waited.

"You're a patient man," I said. "I know you wanted to get an early start, and it's past ten." Inwardly, I admitted that if it had been John's father, my patience would have worn thin.

We drove in silence until John turned onto the freeway. I said, "Dad's message is burning a hole in my purse." John was passing a car and did not respond. "'Have a good life.' What do you suppose Dad is trying to tell me?"

Still preoccupied with the traffic, John said, "Probably just small talk. I wouldn't take it seriously."

"Have a good life." My uneasiness about Dad, and Frank's evasion of the problem, took me back to the time when I had stayed overnight at my brother's. Again and again, I had tried to discuss Dad's depression. Again and again, Frank had changed the subject, visibly unwilling to face the problem.

Another incident flashed on the screen of my memory. One afternoon, Dad had disappeared from the cottage. Finally, Amy and I drove into town to search for him. At the city limits, catching sight of his tall figure, Amy pulled over to the curb. I got out of the car and, running to keep pace with my father, called to him, "It's almost dinner time. Aren't you hungry?" At first, he seemed not to hear. I called to him again.

He stopped, shook his head, and said, "You don't understand. Why should I go back?"

I could think of only one answer: "Because we love you, Dad."

He laughed scornfully. "Love! You talk about love," and began to walk again.

I tried a conciliatory tone. "Remember all the good meals we've shared."

"Oh, sure. A few snacks." He shrugged and stepped up his pace, past our parked car, and past a woman who stopped and stared.

I was breathless. "Please wait, Dad. Please wait."

Amy was cruising beside us. "Come on Grandfather. Let's go home."

She stopped the car. Begrudgingly, Dad got into the front seat. I followed into the back seat and reached over to lock his door.

"We were anxious about you Dad," I said. "I'd never leave you and make you worry about *me*."

Without warning, my father unlocked the door, flung it open, jumped out of the car and shouted, "God damn it. You just don't understand."

"Let him go, Mom," Amy said. "Let him fight it out alone."

Soon he disappeared into the dusk. Fearing he might stumble and fall, I persuaded Amy to follow him on foot. From the car, I watched him slump down onto a park bench. Amy sat down beside him, put her arm around his shoulders and kissed him. He waved his arms wildly and shouted something I could not understand.

A policeman stopped to remind me the time on the meter had expired. Extracting a coin from my purse, I said, "My father refuses to come home."

"I'm sorry, ma'am," the officer said. "I have no authority to force him." He turned and walked away.

I needed help, and there was no help. I felt deserted and alone. I considered phoning Frank, but at a distance, how could he help?

Amy returned to the car and said, "Grandfather's promised to take a taxi home. We may as well leave."

When we reached the cottage, Jan, who had come on vacation, asked, "Is this what it means to be senile?"

I hated the word, but could think of no other way to describe her grandfather's condition.

A half hour later, a car door slammed. In a moment, Dad was in my arms, weeping and asking forgiveness.

Forgiveness was easy, but living on top of each other in the cottage, with no privacy, was becoming increasingly difficult. Night after night, Dad's mumbling kept me awake. Morning after morning, I struggled to face the day. One night, close to hysteria, I escaped to the car with a blanket and pillow. John followed. Insisting on taking Dad back to town, he said, "You'll get sick if this continues. The girls and I need you."

"Have a good life!" Parking in front of The Haven, John brought me back to the present. I thought, "The girls and John need me. Dad needs me. How can I divide myself? 'Have a good life' . . . 'Have a good life.'" How could I under the circumstances?

As John turned off the ignition, I began to cry. He pressed my hand. "I'm sorry your father gives you such a hard time. He's a stubborn old man."

"Each time I suggest that he get an antidepressant," I said, "he laughs and says that on his last visit, the doctor reported, 'You're in good health. Do you want to live forever?'"

"Your father's a stubborn old man," repeated John.

"That's the hardest part—he calls all the shots," I said, dejectedly. "And I'm trapped."

The Haven was waiting, like a mother holding out her arms to shelter us, offering us a weekend of freedom.

Home again, on Tuesday, I found Dad still distraught, still

threatening to leave town. Again the doctor diagnosed it as hardening of the arteries. I clung to hope for my father, as I recalled that some elderly people were no longer considered "senile," but were found to be suffering from health problems of another nature that could be corrected or at least helped.

The doctor repeated, "Your father has hardening of the arteries."

"Does that mean he will become. . . ," I hesitated, faltering with the word, "incompetent?"

The doctor's answer shook me. "That depends on how long he lives."

The significance of his words forced me to phone my brother again. "The doctor says Dad's actions are caused by hardening of the arteries—that eventually he could become incompetent. I guess we have to face it—Dad's senile."

A moment of silence was interrupted by Frank's gasp. "Hardening of the arteries. My God! Until now that never got through to me."

Chapter Seven

As a child, I used to receive letters from my father on his business trips, his sentences interspersed with clever sketches as substitutes for words. As I approached adulthood, his letters elaborated on current events or religious issues; they stirred my thinking and awoke me from apathy. All through the years, Dad's letters were to be treasured.

But I began to dread his carbon-smudged messages that came to The Haven: "I'm going away soon." His cry for help, "I don't know what I'm going to do." His veiled threat, over a shaky signature, "Have a good life."

Although my father's sight was deteriorating rapidly and he was becoming more insecure, more confused, and more disoriented, it was clear he had not lost his ingenuity. When the ribbon mechanism on his typewriter failed, he turned out letters without a ribbon, using a carbon between two sheets of paper, producing only one copy. Each letter I received was a carbon.

At first I ignored the plea that became repetitious: "Come home soon. I've given you power of attorney. You have every moral and legal right to handle my finances."

That my father was eager to relinquish the freedom to manage his money seemed incongruous, so I took each message with a grain of salt until John phoned that Dad was carrying three hundred dollars in his wallet, which he frequently misplaced. After he lost his wallet again and frantically summoned John to help find it, I decided to go home.

As I drove homeward, I tried to adjust to the idea of managing my father's financial affairs. Throughout the years, he had been so alert. I never dreamed of his mind deteriorating. Now I feared he might he mugged and robbed. I worried that he might overdraw our jointly-owned checking account, making me responsible for the discrepancy.

As I sought legal counsel, I decided to set up guidelines. First, to relieve me from some of the burden, my brother would need to assume half of the financial management. Frank agreed.

"This emergency must never separate you and me," I said.

Frank's answer was a comfort. "Of course, it never will."

But loneliness dogged my steps when the lawyer made it clear that the major load must be mine, since my brother resided out of state, and urged me to become Dad's guardian. Another lawyer informed me that a guardianship would entail reporting to the State, and was unnecessary since my father had given me power of attorney. Then I decided on my second guideline: I would assume no responsibility that was a legal one—only a moral one, to be determined solely by me.

These and other guidelines, as time passed, were to become a supportive point of reference, giving me security as stressful circumstances arose, when confusion was overpowering, when sudden decisions had to be reached, when a feeling of guilt threatened to take the upper hand.

Often people said to me, "Of course you take care of your father—he took care of you as child." Or, "Of course you take care of him—because someday you may be in his condition." Then guilt hung over me like a shroud.

I began to wonder: Were either of these reasonings valid? Did they strengthen me for my responsibilities? On the one hand, I had not asked to be born; my mother and father wanted a child and enjoyed taking care of me. On the other hand, I might never be in my father's condition, but even if this happened someday, must I pay for it in advance?

I decided that the only way to stop shadow-boxing with guilt was to determine *why* I was assuming the care of my father—the *real* reason, no matter what it might be, not a reason handed to me by others, but the *truth*. For me, the truth was twofold. First of all, I was taking care of Dad because I loved him. Second, and this was not easy to admit, I was assuming the responsibility because no other person was available.

After dividing my father's savings equally between my brother and me, I dreaded facing Dad with the fact that this had been accomplished. The depressing scene, as I opened the apartment door, was not conducive to breaking the news. Seated at the table typing, Dad was clothed in old trousers with cigar burns, a thermal undershirt that was soiled, and worn house slippers. He was surrounded by wads of typing paper. He ran his fingers through his hair—so long that it curled at the ends. His face was prickly with several days' stubble. His words were as pathetic as his appearance, "I just can't seem to write." The page in the machine proved it, for the same paragraph had been typed and retyped.

I plunged into the problem. "Dad, I received your letters . . . ," and awaited an answer. He snuffed his cigar butt in a saucer and looked bewildered.

"You urged me to come home to handle your money," I said. "I took care of it today."

He looked startled. "What do you mean?"

"You begged me to manage your affiars. You gave me power of attorney. I've made arrangements to take care of your bank account."

"Then how can I pay the rent?"

"Frank will send the rent to Mrs. Martin, then she'll give you the receipt."

He began to pace the floor. "But supposing I run out of money for food?"

I tried to appear calm, but my heart was pounding. "You'll have all you need because I'll check your wallet regularly and replenish it with one dollar bills—so you won't need to figure out the denominations."

He continued pacing, stopped suddenly in front of me, pointed his finger at me and shouted, "You can't know my needs. Nor can Frank. He's too far away."

I hoped that if I left he might settle down for the night. As I reached the door, he shouted, "I want my money. You have no right to keep it." His shouts followed after me.

The nightmare was never-ending. I began each day dreading to answer the phone and was haunted constantly by my father's words to the operator: "I'm half blind. This is an emergency. I need to reach my daughter." I braced myself for his demand, "You must return my money. My wallet is empty." I felt like a thief when he shouted, "You have no right to my money. I earned it." When he refused to listen to reason. I hung up. Never before had I resorted to that.

No longer was there humor in Dad's quip, "I'm normally abnormal." Repeatedly, he attached to our door a note that read, "I have no food." He returned to our porch the groceries I gave him, phoned Social Services that he had no provisions, and showed a wad of bills in his wallet and an almost-empty cupboard to the caseworker who visited him. Investigating, she discovered he was eating heartily at the restaurant. Another caseworker reflected, "He's so ingenious. It's almost as if he's the one who is normal and the rest of us aren't."

Over and over, even at one o'clock in the morning, Dad bombarded me with questions: "Has Frank paid the rent?"—though the receipt lay on the table. Or, "Has the electric bill been paid?"—and although I answered, "Of course, otherwise, you'd have no lights," he repeated the question. Again and again, he insisted that I watch him count out the bills in his wallet and report in detail the state of his finances. When he sent for me in the early morning hours, I cried from fatigue and desperation. "If you keep this up, Dad, I'll have a stroke at your feet."

"Even when he apologizes," I told John, "he seems unaware of the stress I am under. It's almost as if he's had a lobotomy."

To Amy, home for a weekend, I said, "If only I had discussed your grandfather's finances with him before I took complete charge. The sudden change has been too drastic for him."

"Don't blame yourself, Mom," Amy said. "He couldn't have remembered even if you had talked to him in advance."

John agreed. "Even if you had warned him, the Old Man would have been upset."

Dad was becoming an obsession. His demands became my preoccupation. His needs blocked the needs of my family. The monster Guilt made me certain I had robbed him of his independence.

The night when I put on a "style show" for him and modelled some new clothes, it was difficult to believe that my father had ever behaved abnormally. He stroked the material again and again, and said, "I'm glad you bought something new." On another occasion, as he was about to leave our house, he kissed me goodnight, started toward the door, then turned to me and said, "I'm sorry for the trouble I've caused you." Often when I left his apartment at night, he stood at the door with the porch light on, waiting until I called that I had reached the street safely. In these brief moments when he seemed normal, I felt abnormal, as if I had dreamed the unreal turn of events.

But they were not a dream. One morning, when I opened the front door, I saw a bent figure pacing back and forth along the sidewalk. He carried a closed umbrella upright. Fastened on it was a hand-printed sign: "AVIS TOOK ALL MY MONEY." Every time a car passed, my father turned the sign in the direction of the occupants. When school children approached, he pointed to the sign. When a man walked by, he stopped him and reported loudly that his daughter had taken his money, then resumed his trek back and forth. At last he paused, removed his jacket, tossed it on the grass, then began to pace again in yellowed undershirt and sagging trousers.

Suddenly he stumbled. I ran to him, touched his arm and said, "I'm afraid you'll fall Dad. You are tired. Let me take you home so you can rest."

He shook his fist. "What do you care? You have my money."

I tried to steer him toward his apartment. "Please! Please, Dad, go home."

He shoved me away and shouted, "How would you like it if I picketed the bank? Or the church?" His eyes were deep-set in a face that was haggard; his gnarled fingers tightened on the handle of the umbrella, pointing it at me.

I escaped when Amy called me to the phone.

A woman's voice said, "How can you mistreat your poor old father?"

"Who are you?" I asked.

"That doesn't matter. Why don't you take care of your father?"

My voice shook. "I do take care of him. You just don't understand."

She continued. "I feel sorry for him. "You're his daughter and you ought to. . . ."

I interrupted, trying to restrain my tears. "If you aren't courteous enough to give your name, then I shall consider this a nuisance call."

She hung up.

The phone rang again; this time I recognized the voice of Mrs. Martin. "Did you see what your father is doing?"

"Yes, I saw him," I said, close to hysteria.

She continued in a tone that was patronizing. "Why don't you give the poor old man his money? It belongs to him."

That's impossible," I said. "He carries large sums in his wallet and keeps losing it." I was living in a glass house and longed to escape from neighbors who were making my business theirs.

The amusement in Mrs. Martin's voice made me cringe. "Who would have dreamed he'd picket you!" Then she laughed. "You know, I think it's kind of cute."

Chapter Eight

Mrs. Martin didn't think it was "cute" the next day when Dad hung signs on the front door of his apartment. One sign read, "Old people should be shot," and another stated, "I don't want to live." She didn't think it was "cute" when her other tenants complained.

Dad discovered still another way to publicize his convictions. He called the *Journal*, expressed his views on discrimination against the elderly, agreed to be interviewed, and allowed his picture to be taken.

Frank cursed over the phone after receiving the article picturing the craggy old man with long hair—a forlorn contrast to the well-groomed retiree in the news five years before, a dismal change in the headline and copy:

MAN FINDS OLD AGE LONELY, BITTER EXPERIENCE

> Sometimes on cold winter nights, he can't get to sleep. When that happens he puts on his only suit, dons a faded gray topcoat, and walks out of the house.
> As he passes the creek, he thinks seriously of throwing himself in. When you are old and alone it often comes to that.

The article said that his dilemma was one of utter dependency, and went on to report that his son Frank had control of his finances, providing for his food, rent, and other needs (omitting my name from the story, at the request of a friend). My father was quoted as saying, "If a man's been independent all his life . . . and then all of a sudden is told he can't handle his own affairs, it comes as quite a shock."

If my name had appeared in the feature, no doubt readers of the *Journal* (some of them old, alone, and anxious) would have stormed me with letters and phone calls, for they began to fill Dad's mailbox with letters of sympathy, sent him cash and religious tracts, and the brand of cigars the article had said was his favorite. A family with fifteen children invited him to a real country dinner, with pork from their own hogs.

After a religious fanatic came with his son who sang a piece he had composed, I said, "Serves you right, Dad, for calling the paper."

My father smiled sheepishly.

I said, "From here on, I won't ask, 'How are you today?' instead, I'll ask, 'Who's beating a path to your door?'"

A letter to the Editor appeared in the *Journal*:

Where could there be a more worthy person than Mr. Yale to help in his older years—and make it a gesture of respect of someone caring from the heart. How can we possibly ignore the dignity he deserves?

Nor did the younger generation ignore Dad's plight, for one afternoon a delegation of elementary school children appeared at his door bearing a lopsided cake they had baked themselves. Announcing they had adopted him as their grandfather, they presented Dad with a "certifecket" of citizenship to their Thankful Town, U.S.A. He had no choice but to accept the honor graciously, but what could be more ironic than to have citizenship to a town named "Thankful" forced upon a man with grievances so widely publicized? What could be more poignant, under the circumstances, than to receive letters composed with childish innocence, such as:

Please come to Thankful town. Ours is a lovely, loving world, and we want to make you so happy that when you wake up in the morning you'll feel like skipping.

Dad was terrified about accepting the invitation. He asked me, "What on earth will I talk about?" Begrudgingly, he let me transport him to the school.

As I guided him gently by the elbow, a child ran to him in the playground and called, "Oh, Grandpa Yale, you came!" Other children tagged after us to the classroom where Thankful Town flourished. They seated him in a big chair, brought him cookies and candy and put them in a paper bag, and begged for stories of the "olden days." As a child climbed onto Dad's lap, he timidly began to tell of his boyhood when there were horse-drawn carriages instead of automobiles and of his father's grocery where crackers were stored in a barrel. Soon Dad became so engrossed in storytelling that he forgot his fears, called his enchanted listeners his "new family," squeezed a child's arm three times, and said, "That means 'I love you.'"

But my father's victory over self-doubt was short-lived, for soon the letters, the phone calls, and the invitations to dinner began to wear upon him. Soon it became clear that he could not cope with the publicity that had sprouted from the seed he had planted when he phoned the newspaper. He became more confused, more frustrated, and less able to relate to strangers who tried to befriend him—even to people he knew.

Later, I discovered his pocket diary with poignant entries that expressed his feelings of helplessness. "Television dead, can't get repairman. . . . Can't see to read much. . . . Honey Jane came today. . . . Henry called about men's breakfast club, but didn't offer to take me. . . . Frank phoned. . . . I don't want to be an emotional problem to my children. . . ."

Day after day I saw him in the park, a lonely figure on a bench, with fading sight, watching the children at play. In his diary was a touching note: "Today I sat in the park. Mr. Winters stopped and spoke to me." Sometimes he carried his blue satchel to the bus stop, but he never boarded the bus. Sometimes when his porch light was on all night I knew he must be pacing the streets until the police took him home. (Mrs. Martin fretted about the light bill.) The role of parent to my father was becoming incredibly difficult.

Sometimes John and I took him out to dinner. Sometimes John took him alone and patiently guided him in and out of the restaurant. Dad always made a point to express his gratitude, but when he reached his door, he would always shake his head and say, "I just don't know what I'm going to do."

Invariably, whenever I returned home from an errand, I would find a message thumbtacked to our door:

> You have created a major crisis by not paying the rent and by not returning all my assets to me personally.
>
> Your father
>
> carbon copy to landlord

o   o   o

You can't KNOW ALL of your Father's NEEDS. By YOUR refusal to return HIS money YOU are destroying YOUR Father's life.   2 a.m.

o   o   o

RETURN
all of my MONEY,
Or do YOU want me to picket the bank
and the Church?   6:15 p.m.

o   o   o

YOU have WON
I am LICKED
I am tired of isolation, frustration,
utter loneliness. I hope you get
a lot of good from my money.

Close to the breaking point, there were times when I stormed, "Take back your money, Dad. I don't want it. Take it and handle your own affairs. Buy your own groceries. . . ."

Then he would look bewildered and say, "But I can't do that. . . . I can't see."

I threw myself into his arms weeping and begging his forgiveness.

He always answered, "There's nothing to forgive, Honey Jane. I don't want you to have any feeling of guilt. I've told Frank repeatedly that you're doing a good job."

A bank officer phoned, upset because Dad had come to his office, pointed his finger at him and demanded his money. He said it was time I committed him.

I replied, "I won't try to keep the bank from signing a petition, but I won't sign one for them and go through the emotional experience of a hearing. The bank must take care of its own problems. I have enough of my own."

The picketing continued in various forms. Sometimes Dad would tap on the window of our porch with his umbrella, shouting, "Avis is a Christian. She took all my money." One night he stationed himself on a bench beside the door. When he refused to leave, I called the police, hoping an officer might persuade my father to go home. The policeman who came urged, "Mr. Yale, let me help you back to your apartment."

Dad was complacent. "That's not necessary. I'm comfortable here." Then, as if he were the host, he calmly introduced us all: "This is my granddaughter, Amy, and my son-in-law, John. And this is my daughter, Avis. She took her poor old father's money."

The officer whispered to John, "Turn on the porch light. He'll soon get tired of the glare and go home."

John did so, but after we disappeared into the house, Dad twisted the bulb, extinguishing the light. He left an hour later.

Amy giggled. "Probably he had to go to the bathroom."

Mrs. Martin, returning from Florida, had received a copy of the news article, and was offended by the reported description of Dad's apartment: "A striped towel is knotted around a leaky pipe under the bathroom sink."

Soon we learned that Mrs. Martin didn't think that was "cute." She sent word that my father must move.

Chapter Nine

I could never adjust to the tap . . . tap . . . tap of my father's
umbrella on the windowpane; to his shouting, night after night, as
we tried to settle in the living room after dinner; to his emotional
outbursts when I tried to persuade him to go home; to his reply,
"I changed my mind," when I reminded him he had begged me
to handle his finances. His tapping and shouting could be heard a
block away. When the phone rang one evening, I went upstairs to
the extension, hoping to find peace and quiet there. Even from
that vantage point, Frank (who was calling) could hear tap . . .
tap . . . tap. "Avis is a Christian." Tap . . . tap . . . tap . . . "She
took all her father's money."

"Dad phoned me at 2 a.m. yesterday," Frank said, "so I'm
shutting off our phone when I go to bed. Dad said to me, 'I don't
see how Avis can take it when I tap on her window.' I asked,
'Don't you think it's time you quit badgering Avis?'"

The sound began again: tap . . . tap . . . tap . . . tap . . . tap
. . . tap.

"I wish Dad wouldn't do that," Frank said.

As our conversation continued, I became aware that Frank
was unimpressed by Mrs. Martin's demand that Dad move. He
insisted, "She won't throw an old man out on the street."

"Don't count on it," I protested. "She assumes he can live

with us, but he's too feeble to manage our stairs to the bedroom and bath."

Frank repeated, "She won't evict an old man."

Ignoring my brother's stubborness, I said, "I think I have an answer to the problem. I just learned of a nurisng home with a vacancy, where Dad would have some social life and a therapist to work with his abilities. If you'll come this Saturday to take him, he can be admitted at once."

Frank volunteered to think it over. He seemed unconvinced when I said it was impossible for me to transport Dad there by myself.

I was bursting from the pressures. "We're fortunate to find a good facility, because the doctor says most nursing homes won't accommodate a patient who is ambulatory, especially one with an emotional problem. I'm sure Dad's friend Harry would help you take him to the home."

It would have been a comfort if Frank had shown more concern for the effect Dad was having upon me. It would have strengthened me if he had offered to come without my urging. When at last he sent word he would arrive on Saturday morning, and needed to bring his wife Betty along with him, I wondered if his reluctance stemmed from the expense of the trip, from facing the placement of Dad in a nursing home, or both.

After Amy and I met the plane, we had a family conference over lunch before Dad was scheduled for a chest X-ray at two. Betty said she had not wanted to come as this was a family matter for us, but that Frank had insisted he needed her support.

As we parked at the curb in front of our house, Dad appeared carrying his umbrella. Attached to it was a sign: "My children took all my money." He stared at Frank as he got out of the car and asked, "Who are you? I don't know you."

For a moment, Frank appeared to be in shock; then he put his hand on Dad's shoulder and said, "It's Frank. Your son."

I felt sorry for Frank, but I could not stop the thoughts that tumbled one after the other in my mind. How would Frank have stood up under the pressure if he had been exposed to Dad's picketing day after day? How would he and Harry persuade Dad to go to the hospital for the X-ray . . . then to the nursing home? I made a decision. Transporting Dad to the home must be Frank's responsibility, not mine.

Amy and Betty and I watched from the window as Harry and Frank helped Dad into the front seat of Harry's car. Two hours dragged by. The fall night was deepening when an aide called from the nursing home. She said, "I've never seen anyone as frightened as your father. He ran off into the woods, and the police are trying to find him." Too distressed to continue our vigil at home, we joined Frank and Harry. As they waited, people in the neighborhood, accustomed to patients running away, had offered their sympathy and the sustenance of coffee and cookies.

In pitch darkness, there was the fragrance of the first frost, and as the dry leaves crackled under our feet, a feeling of terror. Dad seemed far away, lost somewhere in the night. Perhaps he was lying on the ground, injured or dying in the dark, alone.

"It's as if they were hunting an animal," Amy said. "Some things are worse than death. What has he got to live for anyway?" She began to sob, then burst out suddenly, "Die, Grandfather, die."

When the police discovered my father, safe but weary, they could not by law force him into the home unless, after an examination by two doctors, the court had declared him incompetent.

Frank said, "Anyway I wouldn't want to force Dad to stay. Besides, I got a glimpse of some of the patients and they looked heavily sedated. I would resent their doing that to Dad."

I thought, "Frank has no conception of what it's like to cope with Dad. He needs round-the-clock supervision and professional care."

Slumped in the car seat, Dad begged to be taken home. After he had gone to bed, we had another family conference. Clearly the experience of seeing Dad picket us, and his escape into the woods, haunted Frank. My brother was eager to catch the first plane in the morning.

"But this is destroying Mother," Amy said. "She needs you. Can't you stay until tomorrow night?"

Frank was visibly reluctant. In deep thought, he paced the floor, pulling up his trousers, tightening his belt, until at last, he said, "All right. You're my favorite niece, so I'll do it just for you. I'll change my plans, but I must take the plane tomorrow night without fail."

Amy frowned. She said, "Uncle Frank, I just hope you won't regret it someday, because you didn't find a way to put Grandfather into a home where he'd have care that's professional."

Chapter Ten

For the first time in my life I was afraid of my father. Even his blue satchel frightened me, for it symbolized his threat to go away. Constantly, I was working in the dark, wondering what he carried in the bag to support his fantasy about leaving town. When my curiosity got the better of me, I opened the satchel and found at first glance what seemed to be insignificant: a pair of socks, two folders of matches with advertising on them, a safety pin, bits of paper, and a ballpoint pen. Then I opened a folded paper and discovered a gun permit issued by the local police department.

Angrily, I faced the Chief of Police. "It's incredible that an elderly man, known to be emotionally unstrung, would be issued a permit for a gun."

The Chief was calm. "If a person who has never committed a felony asks for a permit, we have to issue it."

But I was not calm. While I suspected my father's intent was to harm himself, not anyone else, there were other risks I did not enjoy contemplating.

What might my father do accidentally, if he became upset with Amy, as he had recently?

She had said, "Look on the bright side, Grandfather. Why don't you tell me the things you have to be thankful for?"

Sarcastically, Dad had named two: A comfortable apartment and his family. Later, he phoned Amy. "I can't sleep because of what you said."

As she felt the old rapport slipping away, Amy was crushed. "She feels bad," I told Dad over the phone.

"I'm sorry," he said, "but she must learn to listen to old people."

"She's too young to understand how you feel, Dad. Don't you think you're expecting too much?"

Then my father escaped into confusion, launched off on a tirade about his money, and said he could never depend upon a set amount from Frank.

"Just ask him for what you need," I said.

"Oh, put me away," Dad said abruptly and hung up.

At a church bazaar, a woman confronted me. "Did you know your father came in last night while we were setting up our displays? He told everyone that you had taken his money."

I was shocked and wondered if people believed my father's story. A friend, Flo Carson, assured me that most people understood. Thereafter, whenever I attended a church service, I braced myself for Dad to appear with his umbrella and sign. I imagined him marching down the aisle turning the sign this way and that during the first hymn. But he never carried out his threat to picket the church or the bank.

Nights, when I feared that Dad might again picket the house, I hid the car on another street to mislead him into believing I had gone away. Weary of going out at midnight to recover the car, I accepted Flo and Bruce Carson's offer to keep it in their backyard.

The Carsons never deserted me. Often they sustained me over a cup of tea, as I unloaded my distresses, as I tried to sort out the dilemma, as I stumbled through my responsibilities. Without their support, the load would have been overwhelming.

Once Dad phoned and said, "You're playing games with me. After I had supper at the restaurant tonight, I stood outside and told people you had taken my money."

Henry Clarke called to deliver the message from Dad, that he planned to see a lawyer.

I said, "My father is fortunate that I'm not the kind of a daughter who would sue him for libel because of the stories he is spreading about town. I hope the lawyer points out two things. First, that Dad hasn't a leg to stand on, because he gave me power of attorney. Second, if he continues peddling these stories, he could wind up with a legal guardian; then he wouldn't be able to enjoy the freedom he has now."

When Dad phoned and whimpered, "Please give me some bread. I'll pay for it," I sent Amy to his apartment with a loaf of bread and a can of soup, urging her not to take the risk of going inside but to leave the package on Dad's porch.

Terror engulfed me whenever Dad stationed himself on the porch, lying in wait for me; whenever the sound of his shouts carried a mile away; whenever I saw him walking toward our house with his cane tapping on the sidewalk.

After a long tirade one night, John pulled the drapes aside, sighed and said, "You can relax now. He's gone."

Looking out, I saw my father walking with his right hand extended as if holding his cane, but his hand was empty.

"It's weird," I said. "I think that's why I'm terrified."

My heart pounded as night after night I peered through the window of his back door to check on his welfare and saw a long strip of paper towelling spread like a carpet along the floor. On it Dad had printed with a shoe polish dauber: "Who has my money? Old people should be shot."

"I can't take it," I told Frank when he phoned.

"Oh, let him have his fun," Frank said. "If printing signs entertains him, let him do it."

But it was not fun for me. I could feel no emotion except anger and *that* made me angry. Sometimes I couldn't even feel angry. Sometimes I thought Amy was right. The experience was destroying me.

Frank continued: "Yesterday, when I called Dad, he said, 'Do you suppose I'll ever see Honey Jane again?' Then he went on to say, 'There's a rift between Honey Jane and me.'"

I said, "Dad will always feel there's a rift between us as long as I'm handling his money."

I tried not to be afraid whenever Dad appeared at the door, but when I invited him to come in, he shook his fist at me and stormed, "I can't trust you and Frank. Neither of you understand my problem." Then he turned to John and shouted, "Avis is handling your finances. Watch out. Someday she'll run off with *your* money, too."

As Christmas approached, watching others shop and plan for the holiday increased my depression. My father had always shared in our festivities. But this year, I dreaded mixing his emotional upheavals with Christmas Day, feared that he might destroy the holiday for Amy and John, and I had wistful thoughts of family celebrations in years past. I had to admit that I was still physically afraid of my father. The decision not to invite him for Christmas was traumatic. Later, when I learned that Mrs. Martin had included him in her family gathering for Christmas dinner, I was glad he had not spent the day alone, but the old feelings of guilt and of longing for the past arose again to haunt me.

Late one afternoon, after Christmas, Dad phoned and begged tearfully, "Honey Jane, please come over after dinner. I want to talk."

With his use of my pet name, my fears evaporated. Our own meal was ready, so I prepared a plate of food for Dad and hurried to his apartment. As I opened the door, the fragrance of tobacco greeted me. His table was loaded with his typewriter and stacks of books and papers. I persuaded him to sit in his easy chair, with the tray of food on his lap, and said, "You'd better eat before the food gets cold."

He began to cry. "It's humiliating to ask Frank for money . . . to have him pay the rent . . . to tell the clothing store to send him a bill for my new trousers. . . ."

"But Frank and I have often asked for your help," I said, "Now it's your turn to ask us."

"I don't know whether I can at my age," he said, sampling the meat loaf and the corn pudding. "It's humiliating."

I laughed. "It's not humiliating to eat my food."

He chuckled, and for an instant the old banter between us seemed to be restored. Then it vanished, and he said, "I just don't want to live."

"That's all the more reason why you need your family."

"But I feel so dependent. I can't go anywhere without asking someone to drive me . . . and today I carried ninety pounds of clothing to the laundromat."

I knew he was mistaken about the weight, but thought it best not to argue. "I'd have taken you in my car if you had asked."

Ignoring my offer, he said, "I feel so isolated. I go to the restaurant every day, hoping to find companionship, but no one ever sits with me."

I thought of the days when businessmen had invited him to their table. "You still have your family," I reminded him.

"But there's nothing to do, no movies, no way to fill the time. I never should have moved back to the memories of your mother. . . ."

"You have us," I repeated as I prepared to leave.

He shook his head. "Maybe you should put me away."

Later, as I sorted some old documents stored in the deposit box at the bank, I discovered an envelope, labelled by my father, "My Last Will and Testament." My hands shook as I read the message inside:

After my death, I want to be cremated and my ashes strewn on the city dump.
(Signed) Thomas R. Yale,
A human reject.

I took the paper home, shredded it, and threw it into the garbage can—where it belonged.

Chapter Eleven

For more than two years, my birthplace next door had stood
unoccupied, lonely, forsaken by its owner who had been moved
to a nursing home. Like its owner, the bungalow was aged, almost
a hundred years old. Despite its modern siding, it was quaint and
old-fashioned, boasting a cement porch with round pillars, a bay
window in one bedroom, and a mulberry tree in the yard. But the
shrubs bordering the front porch were nothing to boast about.
They were tangled, scraggly, and unkempt underneath where
leaves blowing wild every fall had been trapped, testimony to the
sad fact that no one cared.

Last night, a car had parked in the driveway, as if at last the
house was entertaining visitors. When a light appeared in the bedroom, it seemed to awaken from a long sleep. In the early morning, shadowy figures like ghosts of the past, moved about behind
curtains yellowed with age.

A second car parked behind the first. A man got out, pounded
a stake into the grass, fastened a sign to it, the first FOR SALE
sign on the property in over twenty years—an intruder, it seemed
at first, for I was sensitive about the little house where I had first
seen the light of day. Then I had second thoughts that it might be
pleasant to have neighbors again. Perhaps this time a man mowing
the lawn, a woman shaking a dustmop and bringing in groceries,

children playing in the yard.

Like a flash of lightning, a third thought struck me, and like a seed sprouting from a spring rain, an idea grew in my mind, motivating me to phone Frank.

"The house next door is for sale," I said. "It would be a perfect home for Dad. Why not pool our resources for a down-payment and collect rent from him to pay the mortgage install-ments?"

"It's worth considering," Frank said. Though he admitted there was enough in Dad's fund toward a deposit, he refused to make a quick decision, despite the fact that Mrs. Martin was becoming increasingly impatient; despite my embarrassment about not moving Dad as she requested; and despite Frank's fruitless attempt to find a house near him for Dad, so that now no alternatives remained.

I felt helpless. "We must decide soon, Frank. In this prime neighborhood, that house will be snapped up."

Clearly my brother was not worried. "There's no immediate rush. Even if a prospect appears, getting a mortgage takes time."

Day after day, I watched anxiously from our living room window at the prospects going in and out with the realtor. As I watched a man climb onto the roof, I called Frank again, des-perately. "The man checking out the roof looks as if he means business."

The line was silent. Apparently Frank was holding his usual conference with himself. Finally he said, "Sis, there's plenty of time."

Afterward I imagined losing the chance to buy the house and I visualized my father moving in with us. John and I would have to take turns watching round the clock to keep Dad from falling on our stairs. By midnight I was frantic. I phoned Frank and burst out, "I can't remember the good times. They're gone, and they'll never come back. *You* take Dad. I can't handle him."

Frank said, "I'll have to think of something."

In no mood for thinking, I flared back, "If we lose the house

next door, and if Dad has to move in with us, I'll sell the cottage
. . . and I won't try to go on living." I slammed the receiver onto
the hook.

A moment later, I regretted losing my temper, dialed Frank's
number and apologized.

He said, "All right. Go ahead and make the realtor an offer."

The next morning when I phoned the real estate agent, he
admitted that another prospect was considering the house. My
offer was accepted and the bank agreed to a mortgage in my
name, but not in my brother's, because he lived out of state.
Frank sent his half of the downpayment, saying he wanted Dad
to have every possible "creature comfort," including a fan to keep
the bedroom cool in summer. I added the other half of the down-
payment and signed a codicil to my will, protecting my brother
for half the value of the house.

At last I held the key in my hand. I unlocked the door and
walked from room to room surveying the house. My birthplace:
the home of my maternal grandparents, where my mother and
father had been married; where my mother had come to stay
until I was born.

No one had told my father that he was being evicted again,
or that I had acquired the house next to ours. Remembering the
trauma of his previous eviction, I dreaded breaking the news to
him. Instead, I invited him to go out to lunch and tried to ease
him into the idea of moving again.

"How would you like to have me as your landlady?" I asked.

He laughed. "You must be joking."

"No, this is for real," I said. "I've always wanted to own my
own birthplace. When it was put up for sale recently, I bought it
for a rental, and decided it would be a perfect home for you."

He nibbled his sandwich and sipped his coffee.

The silence was uneasy. I said, "You'd be closer to us.
Wouldn't you like that?"

He shook his head. "You know old folks resist change."

"But there are two kinds of old folks," I said, "those who have no one to help them make the change and those, like you, who have a family."

Again he shook his head.

I decided to drop the subject for a time, to throw my energies into cleaning the house, painting the badly scarred radiators, and moving in some of our furniture.

I dreaded showing Dad the rooms, but the longer I put him off, the more upset he became, and the more frequently he appeared at the door. Finally, I invited him in and took him on a guided tour.

"It's much too large," he said. "I don't need two bedrooms."

I showed him the parlor, where he could watch television, with the French doors closed for warmth in winter. I pointed out the bathroom conveniently located near his bedroom, and on the other side of the bathroom, the kitchen. I kept it a secret that I planned to fasten back the draperies and curtains so I could watch him from our house, but I promised to have a phone installed beside his bed and an extension next to his easy chair in the parlor.

On moving day, to keep Dad from underfoot, John took him to dinner while Amy and I helped the movers transport and place his belongings. When John and Dad returned, Dad became too busy finding his way around to complain. Despite his failing eyesight, he soon found his clothes in the bedroom closet, discovered the light switches in each room, raided the new refrigerator for food, and settled down in the parlor to watch television.

With the draperies and curtains fastened back, I had a clear view from our dinette. I could watch lights go on and off like signals: the lamp on Dad's bedside table, the light in the bathroom, the kitchen light when the bathroom door was ajar. There was comfort in the thought that now I could clean my father's house at my own discretion without considering what a landlady might say. No longer need I wonder about anyone's opinion of Dad's quirks. No longer were either Dad or I living in a "glass house."

In moments of stubbornness, my father was still master of all he surveyed. He still called all the shots, and he still spread paper towelling on the floor with the usual hand-printed complaints.

I faced him. "Dad, there will be no more signs. Is that understood?"

He answered with only one word, "Understood," and from then on he never painted another sign.

But he had some new hang-ups. He insisted on barricading the back door with a chair propped under the knob. He always snapped the lock on the front door when he saw me coming. When I called to him to let him know who was there, without a doubt he heard me and recognized my voice, but he scurried away, leaving the door locked.

There was little consolation in blaming this unusual behavior on hardening of the arteries. For me the thought was earthshaking that, for the first time in his life, my father seemed afraid of me. For the first time in my life I felt rejected.

Chapter Twelve

I cleansed the cut on my father's forehead and quipped, "You and babies have something in common; whenever you fall, you relax, so you never break a bone"—an old joke between us. Dad laughed, but I was worried. This was not the first time he had fallen and the police or a neighbor had had to help him home.

When his legs went out from under him, Dad was plucky. But when he took a psychological tumble, he was so depressed that the doctor suggested a prescription, and I agreed to administer it every day.

As the cumulative effect of the medication increased Dad's alertness, he made his way to the variety store, purchased a pad of yellow paper and a marking pen, struggled all evening until midnight writing and rewriting a letter to Frank. The following day he showed me the finished letter that thanked Frank for the things he had done and added, "Your sister watches me like a hawk. She and John take me out for Sunday dinners when I have chicken with all the fixings and chocolate pie."

Frank promised to answer the letter. When no reply came, I urged him to write soon, so I could put his letter on Dad's table as a reminder that Frank cared. The letter never came.

The longer my father stayed on the medication, the more energetic he became, and the more determined he was to go to the restaurant by himself. To reach the first corner, he worked out a scheme of counting the paces from the house; sometimes losing count, he retraced his steps and started over again.

There were five blocks, one of which was hazardous because of heavy traffic of high school students. "I'm afraid Dad will be hit," I told John. "To protect drivers as well as himself, he shouldn't go out alone." I could think of no other way to accomplish this except to hide my father's street clothes.

Some days Dad was content in the house, clad in his pajamas and bathrobe, socks and slippers, carrying my mother's picture and his wallet in his bathrobe pocket. He wore all of this clothing to bed, despite my protests that the slippers and socks cut off his circulation.

I could depend on him staying indoors when he was in his pajamas. But soon he demanded that I produce his street clothes. Forgetting that people never came, he complained, "If anyone calls on me, I'll be embarrassed to have them see me in my pajamas."

Refusing to give him his suit made me feel as if I was stripping him of his dignity, robbing him of a sense of personal worth. Sometimes his request sounded so reasonable, I thought I had dreamed that his mind had deteriorated, that he could no longer go for walks alone.

To fill his time, I tried to persuade him to listen to the daily news, but this no longer fascinated him, nor did the Talking Books for the blind provided by the library. After years of reading, my father seemed unable to adjust to "listening" to a book.

I began to dread his voice on the phone: "I'm sorry to bother you . . . but it's an emergency. . . ."

I tried to sound matter-of-fact, but my "Hi, Dad" seemed phony.

Hesitantly, he continued. "I didn't want to call you, but someone has taken my clothes."

I tried to explain, "Even if you had your street clothes, it's not safe for you to go out by yourself, because you've fallen."

He seemed not to have heard me. "But without my clothes, how can I go to the restaurant?"

I was driven to drastic measures. "You can't wear your trousers, Dad, because they smell of urine."

"Then there's nothing for me to do but to go to bed," he said, and hung up.

An hour later, the phone rang again. "I was afraid I might awaken you," Dad said. "What am I to do without my clothes?" Becoming desperate, I repeated the old arguments until they seemed like excuses, not reasons; and when at last I hung up the receiver, I was as exhausted as if I had done a day's work.

On more than one occasion, Dad accused me of keeping him a prisoner. He phoned the police often—one day, ten times. The officers who came agreed it was hazardous for him to walk the streets alone. The police chief told me bluntly that my father was my responsibility, not his department's.

The more medicine I dispensed, the more alert Dad became. One morning, I found him in bed, conjuring up ways in which to manage by himself, such as cooking his own meals. He had left an open flame on the stove. Later, he begged to go marketing, but it was icy and treacherous underfoot, and I was nursing an injured leg. He insisted he was out of peanut butter. After he had consumed almost an entire jar, I had hidden the larger container and doled out smaller quantities. It was heart-rending to watch him trying to take care of himself, and frustrating to realize that I dared not cooperate.

I had no recourse but to discontinue the medication. Little by little, as its effect began to diminish, my father became confused again and shrank into a subdued little man who stared into space from his easy chair. As I watched the transformation, I became horror-stricken.

I rushed to the emergency Counseling Center to seek help. "I can't allow my father to use the stove, or to go out on slippery sidewalks, or to overeat," I told a counselor. "By giving him the medication, then taking it away, it's as if I had manipulated him.

What else could I do?"

"You have no reason to feel guilty," the counselor said. "You're not trained to handle the outcome of that kind of medicine."

I had taken the drastic step just in time. A few days later, a call came from Amy, who had married and moved to the West Coast. Her husband, only twenty-seven years old, had been stricken ill and had died.

Amy needed me. So did Dad. There was no easy answer to divided loyalties. There was no other possible decision except to go at once to share her grief. Between John and a neighbor, Grace Burton, whom I had hired occasionally, Dad would have to manage without me.

This was an occasion to be consoled by the fact that my father was forgetful, that to him the calender had little significance, that even though time dragged, he no longer sorted out the hours, the days, the months.

When I returned after a month, Dad seemed not to have missed me, never inquired where I had been or for how long. I volunteered no information, for I had learned when to keep silent.

There were groceries to replenish, meals to freeze, crumbs to clean up from his tray and off the floor. As I spread out the slices of bread, preparing sandwiches for the freezer, Dad shuffled into the kitchen and across the floor in my direction. His eyes had a preoccupied expression. He touched my shoulder and, before I realized what was happening, slid his hand down to my breast. The gesture was so slight, I thought I had imagined it.

The next morning, when I called him to breakfast, instead of going to the table, he turned toward me; shuffling and smiling, shuffling and smiling, as if relishing an intimate secret, he reached out to me suddenly, began to fondle my breast, and simpered, "What have you got that I haven't got?"

The slice of bread in my hand dropped. I ran to the phone in the parlor, called Flo, and began to sob.

After I had recovered from the shock, I felt that if I reported the incident to my brother, he might accuse me of stretching the truth.

Chapter Thirteen

Recent events had provided me with a meaningful slogan: Expect the Unexpected. John and I were on the porch at The Haven when the phone rang. I said, tongue-in-cheek, "I'm prepared for anything—as long as it's unusual."

A voice said, "This is Mabel. Mabel Rush."

Over a period of thirty years, after rooming with Mabel in Newark, the only contact between us had been an annual Christmas card and an occasional letter.

"Where do you suppose I am?" asked Mabel.

"I have no idea," I said, trying not to sound abrupt, but weary of daily shadow-boxing and guessing games.

"I'm calling on your father," she said, then explained that at age seventy-five she had been touring the country, visiting long-lost relatives. Hoping to find us at home, she had stopped by, learned from neighbors where Dad lived, and persuaded Grace to let her in. She planned to drive to The Haven the next day. "It's really nice to meet your father," she said. "We're having an interesting conversation."

"Tell me all about it tomorrow," I interrupted, aware that the long distance charges would appear on my father's bill.

Apparently Mabel was not concerned; she continued, "Would it be all right, Avis, if I sleep on your father's couch tonight?

Otherwise, I'll have to bunk in my van."

Hoping that she did not hear me gasp, I said hesitatingly, "I don't know how Dad would take it."

"Oh, I've talked it over with him, and he says it's all right." Mabel hadn't given me much of a choice; she promised to see me the next day.

When I returned to the porch, John awakened from a nap, and mumbled sleepily, "Your father again?"

I shook my head.

John looked puzzled. "What's up?"

Half laughing, half crying, I said, "If I hoped my father would keep his reputation, all is lost. He's shacking up with a woman." As I finished telling about Mabel, I recalled, "She's always had an eye for a possible match. I hope Dad won't make a pass at her during the night."

John, who had been born without a sense of humor, reflected soberly, "He won't. He's too old."

"She said she'd sleep on the couch. It never occurred to me to suggest that she use the front bedroom." The longer I thought about the situation, the more ironic it seemed. "Until now Dad's called all the shots, with his landlady when she wanted his apartment kept clean, with Frank when he tried to put him in a nursing home, with me when I begged him to change into clean pajamas. Now he's up against Mabel who has a will of steel. I wish them both good luck."

That night as I tossed and turned, I kept wondering if Dad was disturbed by the presence of his house guest. I awoke in a cold sweat after dreaming that Mabel went to her car during the night and, returning to the house, found that Dad had locked her out. I decided it was her problem. If that happened, she'd asked for it.

Even counting the proverbial sheep didn't put me to sleep. My thoughts flashed bck to a day when Dad and I had coffee together and ran out of conversation. We discussed the weather twice . . . Amy and Jan . . . John and his prospective retirement. (We had milked these subjects to the teeth innumerable times before.) Then came Dad's inevitable question, "Did Frank pay the rent?" And my inevitable affirmative answer—whether the rent had been paid or not.

Dad sipped his coffee, and finally said, "You know Frank and Betty lived together before they were married?"

"I can't believe it," I said.

"Yes, they did," Dad said with assurance. "I know because I saw them."

Again I disputed the fact, but as Dad continued to insist he was right, I discovered a new subject to break the monotony—trial marriage!

"I'm all for cohabitation," I said calmly, sipping my coffee and waiting for my comment to sink into Dad's consciousness.

He seemed not to have heard me as he picked up his cane and poked at a patch of sunlight on the floor.

No one was on hand to be judgmental, so I strode knee deep into a controversial but interesting subject. "I'm all for trial marriage. Life gets so daily, and only as two people live under the same roof can they discover the truth about each other: the truth about whether she puts the cap on the tube of toothpaste, the truth about whether he hides behind the newspaper at breakfast. . . ." I stopped to catch my breath.

Lost in thought, my father stared at the window with eyes that were sightless, a pitiful figure with loose threads hanging from his terry bathrobe, wisps of white hair on his collar, the neckline of his pajama shirt stained yellow. Even so, he looked distinguished with his long white hair curling at the ends and his soft pink cheeks deeply grooved.

He sipped his coffee, wiped his lips with a paper napkin, and said solemnly, "Would you want *me* to live that way?"

He could not see my face, but I tried to hide a smile. "Sure, Dad," I said, "If you found a nice lady to keep you company, I'd be all for it."

I would never forget that conversation with its combination of pathos and humor, with its blending of another world (his world) into mine. Recalling it, that sleepless night after Mabel's call, I smiled; if news circulated about my ninety-two-year-old father and Mabel spending the night under the same roof, so be it.

The following afternoon, the same Mabel I had known thirty years before pulled into our driveway in her van—the same Mabel except for her grey hair. She was still vibrant, adventurous, and plucky—having travelled alone for ten thousand miles, sometimes sleeping in her van.

"Your father is lonely," she said at once.

His loneliness always followed me like a persistent shadow. "He refuses to answer the phone or the door," I said, wondering if I was attempting to escape from a feeling of guilt.

Mabel seemed to ignore my explanation. "I made him some breakfast—two eggs, toast, and coffee—and some for myself."

I was curious. "How did he get along during the night?"

"He spent the whole night in his easy chair in the parlor, and kept turning on the light and waking me up to check on me."

I laughed.

Mabel continued, "This morning, he ran his hand along the wall in the front bedroom. When I asked what he was searching for, he said he wanted his suit of clothes, so I hunted until I found it in the closet and helped him put it on over his pajamas."

There was no way I could conceal my dismay. "That's a disaster. Now he'll walk uptown and risk falling or being hit by a car."

The phone interrupted. Dad's voice was frantic. "I went to the restaurant for lunch. There's only a dollar left in my wallet. How can I buy my dinner tomorrow?"

"Grace will come over and prepare it," I said. "Meantime, I'll phone and ask her to stop by tonight to help you take off your suit."

He objected, but I reminded him that his suit would get wrinkled. I hoped after Grace helped him, he would be weary from his adventures and settle down in bed.

Clearly, Mabel did not share my concerns, for she appeared unshaken and, shortly after dinner, went to bed in the den.

Later, when John and I retired, I whispered, "Never in the world would I have gotten up yesterday and said, 'Today Mabel Rush, whom I've not seen for over thirty years, will phone me . . . long distance . . . from Dad's house . . . where she'll stay over-night . . . then help him into his street clothes . . . so he'll go uptown alone to the restaurant.'"

John had escaped into slumber, snoring loudly. As I began to doze off, I remembered my slogan, "Expect the Unexpected," and thought sleepily, "Now I understand what my mother used to mean by her quip, 'It's no laughing matter, no matter if you laugh.'"

Chapter Fourteen

The comedy at the high school had done little to lift our spirits, John and I agreed, as we drove home in the cold. Since John was not feeling well, I had offered to drive. The roads were icy, so I drove slowly, and when we reached home, I eased the car in between the mounds of snow in our driveway and locked the garage while John went indoors. I walked carefully along the glistening snowpath, trying to avoid the patches of ice; thought I heard a voice coming from Dad's bedroom; and paused to listen. His window was closed, so I could hear only the sound, not the words. Fearing Dad might be ill, I hastened onto his porch, removed the key from the mailbox, entered the house, and stood motionless in the unlighted room. Suddenly the words broke the silence, enunciated sharp and clear, like a man delivering a speech, accelerating into a pathetic cry. "How long will it take, God, to starve me? . . . How long?

I wanted to run, to escape to our home where the warm glow of a lamp beckoned.

Dad's voice was becoming increasingly louder. "How long will it take? How long? God, you broke all of your promises. Where were you when I needed you? Where are you now?"

The house was warm, but I shivered. Frank was far away, physically and psychologically. I was alone and fearful.

"Who has my money? I used to pray and pray . . . used to believe your promises, God. Now I'm alone . . . blind . . . deaf. . . . How long . . .?"

I ran from the house into the cold, too inwardly frozen to cry.

"What's wrong now?" asked John.

"He's so lonely. I can't stand it. He's crying for help. . . . I'm going back to fix him some milk toast."

"Don't do it," John urged. "It's too late. Go in the morning. He'll only take it out on you now."

"I can't desert him," I insisted. "I've got to go back. It's tonight that he needs me."

Out into the dark, I returned to Dad's living room where I had left a lamp glowing. I listened but heard only silence. I hoped he had drifted into deep slumber, escaping his suffering.

Again the silence was broken, "How long, God? How long will you take to starve me?" He raised his voice. "Can't you hear me? Am I not shouting loud enough? Or are you too busy?"

Trying to drown the sounds, I snapped on the kitchen light, opened the refrigerator, removed a bottle of milk, and slammed the door. Dreading to face my father, I turned on the bedroom light to dispel the shadows.

At his bedside, I bent over him and said, "I came to fix you some milk toast."

He sat up in bed and slid his slippered feet to the floor, his eyes vacant as if the nightmare had faded. Like an obedient child, he followed me into the kitchen, moved the chair from barricading the door, and sat down at the table.

With the patience of one who had nothing to do but wait, he stared into space as I covered bits of toast with warm milk, salted it, and dropped in globs of oleo.

He sipped the milk from a spoon slowly, as if it were a delicacy. I sat opposite him with a cup of warm milk for myself and tried to think of something to fill the gaps before another tirade might start.

"Charles Chaplin's grave has been robbed," I said. "And a

ransom demanded."

My father continued eating without commenting.

"The body of Charles Chaplin has been stolen."

"I didn't know he had died," Dad said.

"About a month ago."

"A strange thing to do, stealing a body."

I searched for another subject. "The coal miners have staged a strike."

There were long spells of silence, interspersed with bits of conversation. After a half hour, I said I needed to go home.

My father carefully tipped his chair under the doorknob and shuffled back to bed. For a moment, I waited in the darkness, but no sounds came from the bedroom. I thought how strange it was that utter loneliness could be dispelled by a "creature comfort" like a bowl of warm milk toast.

Chapter Fifteen

I was two weeks late in tearing April's page from the calendar. May had arrived, there was no doubt, for each warm day teased our yard and Dad's into new life, and kept John and me busy with spring clean-up. Nature's cauldron of fragrant growth, cooking in the sun, stirred by soft breezes, had stimulated my thoughts of days long gone, making me vulnerable and aware that I was hovering between two worlds—my father's and my own. Sometimes I was buried in Dad's world, a No-Man's land, saturated with its frustrations, haunted by its isolation, lost in a maze where I kept searching for some remnant of the sixty years we had shared. Groping for my own world, I heard The Haven calling, and sought in thought its healing promise to renew my weary spirit.

Across the way, Dad's bedroom window was blank, an empty picture frame. From habit, I watched for signals. From somewhere, far off it seemed, I heard John say, "The car is ready now for you to hit the trail."

"But I'm not!" I said, still watching for signs of life next door.

"You've put off leaving long enough," he said. "I'll be coming to The Haven soon. Meantime, even a short change of scene will do you good. Besides, I'm getting nervous to know if the cottage was vandalized last winter." (Clearly the latter was a hoax to get me on the road.)

Suddenly Dad's bedroom window brightened. A picture appeared within its frame: the bedside lamp spotlighting his figure wrapped in blue terrycloth, bent over, groping along the floor for his slippers, forgetting they were always on his feet.

"I'm homesick," I said to John. "You know I always get homesick before I leave."

John laughed. "Silly! The Haven is home, too. You'll feel better after you get on your way."

How could I explain to John, to anyone? The lighted window had triggered my thoughts into a wave of homesickness for the days when my father had been "himself."

"Dad's up," I said. "I'll fix his breakfast before I take off."

I crossed our lawn to Dad's, the dew chilling my feet. "I'm homesick," I repeated aloud, looking to see if a passerby might have overheard. No one was in sight except a neighbor in his car. "I'm so lonely for the old days," I whispered.

As I fitted the key into the lock, I saw Dad shuffle into the kitchen, remove the chair barricading the back door, sit down at the table, and reach into the refrigerator.

I moved quietly and thought, "I can't bear to have him run from me this time, not when I'm going away."

When I reached his side, he quickly closed the refrigeratror, like a child caught raiding it.

"How about a hot breakfast, Dad?" I asked.

He did not answer.

"How about something hot?"

"That would be nice," he said. (I missed the old days when he used to ask, "What gets you up so early?")

While he sipped his juice, I boiled an egg, toasted two slices of bread, and heated water for coffee.

"Smells good," he said, as I set the food on his tray. "Thank you."

Why did his gratitude depress me? Was it the submissive quality of his voice? His subservient attitude? Dear God, had I caused him to feel subservient to me!

I filled my cup and his, "Be careful. It's hot." I brought a chair from the bathroom for myself, thinking, "Dad used to get it for me."

"Thanks for the hot food," he said, engrossed in breaking his toast into smaller pieces.

Then the silence. Oh, the deadly silence! What news could I relate that had not been told the day before, or the day before that? He nibbled his toast, dribbled crumbs upon the tray, and wound his watch. My coffee had cooled enough to sip; as long as I could make it last, there was an excuse to linger.

The day before, I'd risked an argument but persuaded Dad to change into clean clothes (but not to let me bathe him); into an undershirt, permanently stained about the neck from constant wear, now permated with the sweet smell of sunshine from drying on the clothesline; into his flannel pajamas and blue terry bathrobe from which I had trimmed the ravellings; and into fresh socks, after soaking his feet and cutting his overgrown toenails.

Dad bent over his cup. His hair, shampooed the day before, was pure white, the way my mother loved to see it, the part making a pink line in his clean scalp. He had managed to shave a little the night before, missing some stubble that touched the childlike softness of his cheeks. On each side of his face delicate white tendrils, forming uneven sideburns, moved in slow rhythm as he chewed his food.

To prolong my stay, I refilled my cup. Despite the silence, the atmosphere seemed less strained, but far removed from years past when we had aired our views, agreed to disagree, bantered back and forth, and had shared trials that were mutual.

I said, "Yesterday a letter came from Amy, and one from Jan." (I had told him that the day before.)

"That's nice," he said. "Does Amy still work for Jan's husband?" (He had asked that yesterday.)

"Yes. Both girls said, 'Tell Grandfather we love him.'"

In the shadows his face became illumined with a smile. "I love them, too." He broke a corner from his toast. "What have you heard from Frank?"

"He never writes to me anymore."

"Or to me. I'm always interested in Frank and his children."

I clasped my hands beneath the table, partly to keep from exploding about Frank's failure to write Dad, but mostly to hold my one remaining treasure—my father's love. Deep within his lonely, silent world, buried beneath confusion and forgetfulness, remained an abiding love for his grandchildren, and for the rest of us, his family. Of that an old, old man's incompetence could never rob us. Yet sometimes, no matter how I tried, I could not resurrect the old feeling of closeness.

I drained my cup again. Someday I'd wish I had asked Dad to re-tell the stories of his boyhood: of Mother as a girl, of Frank's life and mine as children. What would I long to recall, in case something happened to Dad before I returned? I thought, "He's all I have left of the family I grew up with. I don't even have Frank anymore."

I touched Dad's arm and said, "I'm leaving for The Haven. Grace will get your meals while I'm away."

"What day of the week is it?" he asked, as he reached for a napkin and wiped his mouth methodically, back and forth.

"It's Wednesday, Dad." I cleared the table, stacked the dishes in the sink, and wiped crumbs from his tray.

"What month?"

"It's May."

"How long will you be gone?"

I hesitated. "Only a few days. There's cleaning to do at the cottage, for the summer. Grace will fix your meals."

If it were true that angels resided in heaven, would my mother be watching over him? (I tried to picture her in an angel's robe with wings.)

Leaning over my father, I kissed his soft, soft cheek and whispered, "I love you, Dad."

He raised his face to mine, returned the kiss, and said, "I love you, too."

"I'll leave the door open to let in the fresh air."

At the front door, the fragrances of spring dispelled the stagnant odor of old age.

My father's voice followed me. "Thanks for everything."

I turned for one more look—a long one—to memorize my Dad.

Chapter Sixteen

"Poor old man . . . Poor old man," I recited again and again as I crossed over our lawn to Dad's, stepping up my pace to keep the tray of food hot. The chanting was a disciplinary measure to control my temper, but as usual my control snapped when I reached the door and Dad locked it.

"Poor old man . . . Poor old man . . ." I was not consoled when some said that he could not help his behavior. I had to deal with it. I was not relieved when some said he did not know what he was doing. Months after his picketing, he had threatened to do it again, so he must have been aware of his actions.

"Poor old man . . . Poor old man . . ." Awkwardly, I balanced the tray in one hand, while putting the key into the lock with the other. I had heard of people who became angry with a loved one for dying. My father was dying a little each day. Could this be the reason I became angry with him?

"Poor old man . . . Poor old man . . ." I followed him into the bedroom, my frustration increasing with the feeling of being deserted by my brother as I watched Dad pull the covers over his head. I tried to release the blanket from his fists, but his grasp was stronger than mine.

I kept telling myself not to scream, but I felt like a parent overwhelmed by the misbehavior of a child. I yelled hysterically,

"Why didn't you open the door?"

There was no answer.

I screamed the question again.

He mumbled, "I'm sorry."

I pulled at the sheet and it ripped—a long gash, like the opening of a wound. Angry with myself for becoming angry, I made an effort to lower my voice and urged, "Your food's nice and hot, Dad. Why don't you come and eat it before it gets cold?"

Little by little, I wheedled him out of his hiding place. Removing his cane from its place on the back of the bed, he followed me into the kitchen, pulled a chair to the table, sat down, and said, "Thanks for the hot meal."

I was still shaken from a tumultuous episode of the previous day. Heretofore, my father had always showered daily. Now he was incontinent, made no attempt to bathe, refused to change his nightclothes, until the stench from his body and his stained pajamas was overpowering. Yesterday, I had insisted that he sponge himself off at the bathroom sink.

He kept saying, "But I can't see."

I kept answering, "You don't need to see in order to bathe. You can feel."

Finally, with some hesitation, he had promised to try.

I laid out clean pajamas in the bathroom, left him by himself, but watched through a slit in the doorway. He moistened a washcloth and rubbed it over his face. With no attempt to sponge off the rest of his body, he hung the washcloth over the rack. Without changing his pajamas, he turned toward the bedroom.

I opened the door and called to him, "Please let me help you, Dad." Taking the washcloth from the rack, I began to unfasten his bathrobe.

He grasped my wrist, twisted it, and shouted, "No woman is going to give me a bath."

"Then I'll hire someone else to do the job," I retorted.

He shook his fist in my face. "You have all of my money."

In desperation, I ran home to John and stormed, "I'll never again attempt to give him a bath. Not even if he stays dirty for the rest of his life."

The local Office of Aging must have been psychic, for it gave the Visiting Nurses agency a list of elderly people who needed help, including my father. A nurse from the agency came for an interview, was astonished that Dad was taking no medication, but soon discovered why when she checked his heart and blood pressure and found both were normal.

The nurse urged me to buy sheets that were fitted. (Had she never learned to turn a square corner in unfitted ones?) She insisted that a fire alarm should be installed. I explained that the sound would frighten Dad out of his wits. She assured me that an aide would come twice a week to prepare a hot meal and to do light housekeeping—to be reimbursed by a special fund for persons on a low income. I began to wonder if Dad and I were about to live in a glass house again.

I filled the cupboard with cans of fruit, soups, vegetable juices, and tuna fish; the freezer compartment of the refrigerator with fruit juices, complete dinners, chicken livers, and baked sweet potatoes wrapped individually for snacks. To hide food that Dad might overeat, I put perishables like cottage cheese in the crisper drawer and crackers and cookies in the stove drawer. Beside Dad's tray, I kept a thermos of coffee and one for hot cocoa. In a small jar, I rationed peanut butter, which he liked to eat with a spoon.

I emptied a drawer in the kitchen, labelled it "Message Center," where I would leave instructions for the aide and where the aide could leave notes for me. Beside the phone, I taped an emergency list of phone numbers: mine, the doctor's, and the ambulance service's.

The aide soon discovered why I had to keep quantities of food hidden. She gave Dad a hot meal, prepared enough sandwiches and snacks for overnight, and filled both thermos bottles. After his meal, Dad watched television for a half hour, then returned to the kitchen and raided the refrigerator, depleting the food supply. This happened again on the aide's second visit. She asked to be assigned to another patient.

The second aide was equal to the situation, as indicated by the notes she left in the Message Center:

> Your Dad ate like there was no tomorrow. I washed his hair and trimmed it some, but since I hadn't my hair cutting set along didn't do too well. Will trim and shape it better when I bring my things. I have your note. Thanks. Pat.

• • •

> Everything went fine today. Patient ate well, talked none, but maybe he is afraid of me, as I come at him from all sides, barbering, shaving and such. Poor man doesn't have a chance. Pat.

The moment I opened the door, I knew when Pat had come, for the sweet-and-clean aura and the aroma of tempting foods spoke eloquently of her presence. She spent her own money to buy treats to tickle Dad's palate, brought a fitted sheet from her own linen closet to silence the nurse's complaints, tried to work around Dad's stubbornness, and cheered and supported me when my spirits were low. Whenever Pat was on hand, it seemed as if angels did not reside in heaven, but on earth.

Sensing that I felt deserted, she said, "I just cannot understand why your brother doesn't come for a visit."

"I've begged him to come," I said, "but he insists he can't afford the trip. I felt sorry for Dad when he said he hadn't received a Christmas card from Frank."

As the weeks passed, there were repeated confrontations with my brother: about finances, about Dad's care, about Frank's neglecting to write Dad.

When the funds in my charge began to dwindle drastically, due to costly household repairs, I asked Frank for extra money from Dad's account in his care. Frank sent a check to help with taxes, then refused to send anything over and above the "rent," utility costs, and fifty dollars each month for Dad's food and personal needs. My brother's chief concern was that he might run out of money for emergencies in the future. But I insisted that I could not get a job to support Dad, as well as take care of him, nor could I dip into John's income.

"Don't complain," Frank said. "Betty and I offered to take Dad, but you refused to go along with the idea."

"That's not true," I responded hotly. "When you tried to find a house for Dad near you, I offered to cooperate, but you were unable to find a place so I was forced to move him next door. If he becomes bedridden, I'll need to put him into a nursing home."

Frank's voice was despondent. "Amy hurt me that time she said she'd hoped I'd not regret that I didn't institutionalize Dad." His tone sharpened. "Do you really mean you'd sock him into a nursing home?"

"I'd have no other choice, if he becomes an invalid. I can't possibly lift him. In the meantime, the very least you could do is to write him."

Frank's voice blistered the wires. "I'm no longer your little Frank Yale. Just because you're nine years older, don't think you can boss me as you did when we were kids."

On another occasion, Frank lashed out, "I haven't forgotten the night you called and put me on the spot about buying the house."

One night, my brother phoned Dad as I worked in his kitchen. I could overhear my father telling Frank that I provided good meals, but he complained that I insisted on keeping him clean. "Your sister gets pretty highhanded," Dad said. "She just doesn't understand."

Their conversation continued for an hour, with Dad keeping his tone confidential, without Frank offering me a chance to tell my side of the story. Tongue-in-cheek, I conjectured that although they considered my services unsatisfactory, neither Frank nor Dad had suggested that Frank relieve me of my duties.

To be sure, I was ashamed of the times when I had lost my temper. But from firsthand, everyday experience, I had been enlarging my vocabulary with such words as *incompetence, senility,* and *incontinence,* while my brother knew the definition of these only as they appeared in the dictionary and was all too ready to criticize me.

My guilt feelings began to subside, then, as I reached a decision. Since I was the one assuming the responsibility of my father's care, it was presumptuous of anyone to complain about me. From then on, I was determined to accept no criticism: not from Dad, not from Frank, not even from myself.

Chapter Seventeen

"I'm falling apart," I told John. "Sometimes I find it difficult to think of Dad as my father."

That morning, longing to disappear where no one could find me, I had driven to the shopping center, parked, and slept in the car for over an hour.

Every night, obsessed with my father's problem, I had been sitting facing his bedroom window, until I became so depressed that I was forced to draw the shades. It was an effort to tackle anything beyond daily necessities. When asked to do volunteer work, I shied away from any involvement, no matter how small. The advice to "think of others," as good therapy, fell flat; I *was* thinking of another—my father—and I was saturated with that responsibility.

Returning home from the parking lot, I told John, "I feel trapped, and I feel guilty about feeling trapped. I don't even feel like a human being."

In desperation, I threatened to leave the state, although I didn't mean it. The doctor said, "They'll follow you," without explaining who "they" might be. "Unless he has a stroke or breaks a bone, your father is unlikely to be eligible for skilled care in a nursing home, and no adult foster care facility could keep him from wandering." It became apparent that an ambulatory person who was blind, deaf, and disoriented was not considered ill or disabled, just *old*.

Sometimes to save sanity, I prepared quantities of food for Dad's refrigerator and a thermos of coffee, then disappeared for the day. Periodically, I sought direction at the Mental Health Department, where a counselor, whose mother had been confined to a nursing home, pointed out sympathetically how difficult it is to change roles by becoming a parent to a parent. When I was depressed, she encouraged me to seek interests of my own, and helped me weather burdens that were overpowering. But I learned to examine what I was told with a caustic eye, for not every counseling experience was rewarding.

On one occasion, a counselor asked, "Do you mind if I tape our conversation?"

"For what purposes?" I asked.

"For the use of students in the field," she replied.

Recalling an instance of a student who recognized a taped voice, I decided for the sake of privacy not to be taped. Later I told another counselor, "I wish I hadn't been asked. It's as if someone across the street requested that I leave my shade up while I undressed. If the tape had been made, I'd have felt naked."

"But you were offered the chance to refuse," she said.

Some counselors were on the defensive when I related this experience. They overlooked the fact that on the spur of the moment, I might have agreed to the taping, then regretted it later. They seemed unable to comprehend that I had had enough of living in a glass house.

Sometimes it seemed as if counselors lacked both training and experience in the problems of the aged. In a time of crisis, the local Mental Health Department referred me to a counselor who did not handle problems like mine.

When I was overcome by the feeling that Frank had deserted me, a therapist urged, "Tell your brother you're through." It was a foolish admonition, for had I done so, Frank would have called my bluff, knowing I would never desert Dad.

In a moment of stress, I considered trying to find an adult foster care home for Dad, and even called a director in charge of placement.

"You owe it to yourself to live your own life," she urged. "Again and again, when I talk to relatives of the aged, they have difficulty comprehending this."

"But supposing my father becomes hostile and refuses to cooperate?"

The director's mood changed. "Of course, I can't guarantee they will keep him."

I could picture Dad getting up in the middle of the night, as was his custom, to get a snack . . . searching for the refrigerator . . . awakening his roommate . . . realizing suddenly that he was not at home . . . becoming angry and planning an escapade that would force his release.

I asked, "If that happened . . . then what?"

"They wouldn't keep him," she said. "After all, these foster homes are run usually by couples who have other jobs and hire someone else to be in charge. They haven't time to take care of the unruly."

If I were to make another attempt to place Dad in a care facility, possibly he would respond to medication supervised by professionals. Or perhaps he would become incorrigible, requiring sedation or some other controlling measure. Who could prove it, one way or the other?

A counselor said, "No one else can really decide for you how to feel about your decisions. Your feelings belong to you personally."

The pressures had been coming at me from every direction. Not just my father's increasing disability, but from a series of emergencies in my immediate family. Sorting out my priorities had become a priority in itself: when Amy's husband died, when I rushed to John to the hospital for surgery and visited him daily for a month, and when John discovered that he had cancer and needed regular outpatient treatment.

Despite the cancer, John was living a seemingly normal life. He promised to look in on Dad in between the aides' schedule (by then increased to five days a week), so I could get a respite at The Haven and enjoy the fall colors.

Before leaving, I bought food for Dad in quantities, tried to anticipate the needs of the aides, and prepared instructions for the Message Center including a daily check of the phone, since Dad had been leaving it off the hook.

At The Haven there was a sense of freedom when I awakened and saw the leaves, hanging like green lace, framed in the bedroom window, and looked forward to a day free of pressures. Soon, however, it became clear there was little escape from the burdens I thought I had left at home, such as: when the phone rang late one night and I stumbled through the darkness to answer, saying aloud, "Dad has died and I wasn't with him," discovering then that a wrong number had been dialed; when Frank called, upset by six long distance calls from Dad; when John reported that the young man, hired to bathe Dad, had quit when Dad threatened him with his cane; when Mrs. Emmons, a caseworker at a social service agency, called to ask when I planned to return home. She said Dad's condition had become worse. He was spending most of the time in bed, was not safe alone, and needed care. If necessary, she would take Dad to a facility herself.

On other occasions, I would have hurried home. This time, it was unrealistic to suppose that if I did so, I could stop Dad from phoning Frank fifty times if he wanted to. Nor could I force Dad to let me give him a bath, or to go to a care facility.

One friend kept urging, "Don't go home yet. You need all the reserves you can accumulate for whatever the winter may bring."

Another friend said, "Maybe you should go home. If your father dies alone, you'll feel guilty, as I did after my mother's death."

Terry Brown, a social worker near The Haven, who had befriended me, urged, "Let the Visiting Nurses handle it. They are trained for this kind of responsibility."

A woman with whom I conversed in a laundromat said, "I'll always take good care of my parents if they become disabled, hoping to set the example for my own children to do the same for me."

I replied, "Don't count on that. If your children see you becoming exhausted by assuming your parents' care, they may be unwilling to make the same sacrifice for you."

Again and again, I heard of others with problems similar to mine. One woman placed her mother in a nursing home, then got a job there. Another postponed much-needed surgery to care for her father. A husband and wife, after placing his mother in a home, never left town even for a short vacation. A friend lost his sister from overwork in caring for their mother. A woman told me, "We had twenty years of the care of my mother and now that it's over, I still look back and feel guilty, despite the fact that my husband insists, and I agree, that I did my best." The professor of a college class in Personal Growth said, "In each of my classes, there is at least one person with an aged relative requiring care."

I longed for the courage of a woman who wrote:

> I've taken care of my mother for sixteen years—and she hates it, too. Four years ago, my husband retired early with Parkinson's Disease. He is not able to do much—so perhaps God in his wisdom has shown us that we must accept this and meet our problems a day at a time. We see so many our age who are facing more difficult problems, so we are grateful for our blessings.

"There is no solution to problems of this kind," said a friend. But it would have helped if I could have associated regularly with others who faced similar problems. When I suggested to a minister that a support group be formed, he agreed to the advantages but had no time to organize one, and I did not know how to begin.

One day I phoned the Drug Counseling Center to ask about the side effects of my medicine for high blood pressure. The young man who answered said the medication could cause depression, and asked, "Are you depressed sometimes?"

"Now and then," I admitted. "I am sixty-six years old, have had the responsibility for my elderly father for five years and still feel guilty for leaving him."

"Then you've taken care of your father longer than most people would. How long are you going to continue feeling guilty?"

He was right about the guilt. Sometimes when I said, "I'll not give my whole life to this responsibility," I fantasized that unless I gave up my life for my father, one of our girls might meet with a fatal accident. I was falling apart for sure.

There was scant comfort in the assurance of those who insisted, "God won't give you a burden without providing you with the strength to carry it." But my strength had been sapped, so I countered, "If God does not give me enough strength to care for my father, could that mean that God does not expect me to handle the responsibility?" Some people were embarrassed by the question. Some were frustrated. Some were patronizing. One person replied, "You're attacking my faith."

A counselor in the field of grief, insisting that God had always provided me with strength, said, "Your feelings of distress are natural, under the circumstances."

"That's a good word—'natural'—I'll hang onto it," I answered.

"It's not only a good word, but it's an accurate one," he said.

From then on, I clung to the word *natural* like a drowning person to a raft.

A thoughtful clergyman said he felt answers were not always what we were seeking; that we need to feel people are sensitive to the depth of our search and want to share it with us. He encouraged me by calling my question "legitimate" and by assuring me that my sense of guilt indicated I was faithful.

In the past, how uninformed I had been about the problems of caring for the aged! With chagrin, I remembered trying to help an elderly woman who wanted to leave a foster home. With embarrassment, I recalled her daughter's phone call requesting that I stop interfering.

With a deep sense of loss, I thought of the early days of my father's disability and my brother's assurance that Dad's problem would never separate us. Sometimes the past intensified the loneliness of the present, especially as I thought of the days when my parents and my brother and I were a family; or reminisced about the delights of Dad's annual visits; or remembered wistfully the days when Frank and I, as adults, had been close.

Dad had changed. So had Frank. So had I.

Would I ever recapture the treasured moments I had lost?

Chapter Eighteen

The green "lace" framed in my bedroom window had turned to gold, awakening me to the overwhelming splendor of autumn. Red and orange and yellow leaves blazed in the sunlight; glorified the street, the lanes, the highways; and made life worth living, no matter what ruts or detours lay ahead in the unknown.

Two miles from The Haven, the State Park, deserted by vacationers, had become my retreat. Late each afternoon I parked on the beach, read a book, dozed off in the car, and awoke in time for the Harvest sunset. As the waves washed the shore and the gulls floated overhead, I tried to sort out the debris in my thoughts; day by day, I recorded them in a small notebook:

"Sometimes the only way I can make any sense out of this dilemma, or feel that I can rise above it, is to decide to live up to my best as Dad would want me to do. What other philosophy is there to cling to?

o   o   o

"I feel sure God gave me the little cottage for a haven, so I am trying not to let my burdens spoil the special experience of being here. If anything can heal this hurt, the forest can, with its

107

varied shades of green, and the autumn leaves—gold and orange and red—surrounding The Haven. I never noticed until yesterday how the tall, thick-trunked trees weave back and forth in the wind. I wonder if people who are strong must bend, too, sometimes?

o   o   o

"I have carried the load so long, it's difficult now to sit back and let someone else take my place. I don't know whether it's woman's intuition, or a sixth sense—but something tells me to wait here. I can't help but feel that Dad has other 'errand people' besides me. The road has been so long. So lonely.

o   o   o

"Mathematics and the calendar often depresss me. Dad is now ninety-four. I am sixty-six. With longevity in our family, he's sure to live until he's a hundred—six more years. In six years, I'll be seventy-two! In those six years, what will I have lost because of this situation? Or is there a way to gain? Some way to feel fulfilled along this detour in spite of an experience that's a nightmare?

o   o   o

"If only I could look back someday and feel that Frank and I were close all through these hard times. The price of losing our relationship has been too great. Some nights, sitting alone, I try sending out love-waves to Frank and Betty, to heal the hurts I've inflicted when, under stress, I've lost my temper. I suppose, deep inside, I keep hoping the phone will ring, and they'll 'take me in their arms.' They can't begin to comprehend how lonely their separation has made the task of caring for Dad. Sometimes I think God is keeping him on earth until we can effect a reconciliation. But where do I begin . . .? I want to do my share—yet I long to have Frank and Betty say and show that they care about Dad and me. Unless this can happen, there will always be an emptiness, an incompleteness in this experience.

o   o   o

"Sometimes I lie in bed picturing Dad's isolation, and the pain of it is more than I can bear. He tried to live in dignity. If only he could die in dignity. The deepest cut of all, looking back at all he accomplished, is the fact that he can no longer make decisions and carry them out.

o   o   o

"*Wait* is the most difficult word in the English language. And what one does while waiting—or what one does not do—can be a yardstick of growth. I have had to learn to wait, to 'play it by ear' until my ears have calluses on them. But I hope not my soul. This time, when I do not know what steps to take, it's as if God were whispering, 'Wait . . . I'll handle it.' I suppose, too, in a sense, I am buying time while the agencies decide what should be done. I do not have the wisdom or the strength to carry it out. Will they?

o   o   o

"I strolled on the beach today and watched the waves wash over the sand, and the color of the hills change from autumn blaze to subdued shadows. The sun broke through some of the billowy clouds. A man walked a dog in the sand. Two girls dipped their hands into the water. The sand dunes rose here and there. I tried to memorize the scene; promised myself no one could take it from me; and reached out for God's hand, this time not to steady myself, but to thank Him for these moments when He has not forsaken me.

∘   ∘   ∘

"When I stepped into the sand I left a print. That's what frightens me sometimes—the imprint I've left affecting those around me. Come quickly waves, and wind, and rain, to make the imprints vanish where I have caused a hurt, or led someone astray, or blemished some other life. When the sands smooth out again tomorrow, my second chance will come to make an imprint that may stay awhile and lead somewhere instead of no place at all.

∘   ∘   ∘

"This afternoon I packed my books and drove to the beach, parking where my eyes could travel all along the coast, northward and southward, lined with trees, and at one point a tree standing by itself—a nonconformist like me. The muted colors spoke of an autumn almost gone. (Which was more golden, the sun or the sand on which it shone?) I watched and read, watched and read in the car, fell asleep and awakening wondered what I'd missed while my eyes were closed. I slipped my shoes and stockings off, walked along the water's edge, wishing I had the courage to wade into the frigid lake.

"A lone girl jogged along the beach past me, flung herself upon the sand, and smiled as I approached. We chatted about the mildness of the Indian Summer weather. She said she was doing her practice teaching. I longed to be that age again; her eyes danced—she was too young to know the cares of a citizen called 'Senior.' She said her name, asked mine, held out her hand to clasp mine and said, 'Good-bye.' It was only six o'clock, but the darkness came on suddenly. I threw a dry stick into the car—a memento of the sand, to spark my fire at night.

"Later at the cottage, I realized how important it had been for me to visit the beach, without having to say to anyone that I was going, or why I was going, or when I would return. In that brief moment of self-realization, loneliness did not rear its dreary head. Instead, I felt a comforting sense of being at one with my Self. It may not last until tomorrow, but tomorrow I can reminisce about this feeling, hold it close—and smile!

o   o   o

"The 'guilt trips' always hit hard—those moments when I fight against remembering my impatience with Dad. When I clench my fists against myself for this, I try to recapture the night when I cried in his arms and begged forgiveness, when he held me tight and said, 'Don't, don't! You've no reason to have a sense of guilt.' His pain in that moment was for my suffering, not his own. If Dad could forgive me, then somehow I must learn to forgive myself.

o   o   o

"Sometimes I long to see my mother, to ask her what to do. She was my father's comforter. Now I must take her place, and often I resent the role. Partly because much of the time I don't know who I am supposed to be, or what I am supposed to do with my life at sixty-six. Separating my own life from my father's is almost beyond my stamina—if I have any left. What would my mother say if she were here? She always put my father ahead of herself. Should I too think only of him?

o   o   o

"The old days seem so distant, and I feel so far from my father. A friend assured me the time will come when I'll feel close to Dad as I used to. I wonder. The scars are so deep, so ugly, so forever. I never knew before that being close to a parent could change to being far apart. How could the old rapport, the old ties, the old camaraderie be wiped out as if they had never existed?

112

＊　　＊　　＊

"Hindsight, they say, is better than foresight. So it's important that I use my hindsight to direct my foresight. I provided the best care for Dad that I could when John and I went to spend Christmas with the girls and their husbands. If we had not gone, we'd have missed the last Christmas as a family before Amy's husband died; then the loss would have been doubled!

"Other times when I've been close to a breakdown, The Haven has given me renewal, strengthened me, and made me feel human again. Sometimes the choices for me have seemed against Dad, in spite of all I've tried to do to provide for his needs during my absence. When it's difficult to reconcile myself to the situation, and especially to the decisions I've been forced to make, like an echo out of the past, my father's admonition recurs: 'Find yourself, Honey Jane. Life is too short to waste. Make something of it.' But *how*?

＊　　＊　　＊

"I keep telling myself: 'Make something special of your life, in memory of your parents who dreamed of your becoming an extension of them. But it's important to become your own person.'

"I am an extension of my mother and father. What kind of an extension will I become? I am an individual. A person in my own right. What kind of a special person will I be?

"My father, as I've known him over the years, would encourage me to honor him by centering my attention upon discovering who I am, and in that light, plan on who I might become.

＊　　＊　　＊

"A psychologist, to whom I wrote, replied that my situation posed a difficult question. He said that I had a *right* to survive. Sometimes I wonder!"

Chapter Nineteen

Sometimes I was terrified by the physical and emotional changes I saw in my "mirror." The quest seemed endless as I searched for my Self. I jotted down questions I needed to ask if I were to survive:

1. *Why* do I take care of my father? (An honest answer!)

2. How much of my own life am I willing to invest in his care? (*All* of it? If so, is that necessary?)

3. Do I sometimes have to fight off the sensation that this responsibility is destroying me?

4. Do I often feel as if I am having to choose between my father's life and my own?

5. Do I experience feelings of hostility toward him?

6. Do I ever wish I did not have this responsibility?

7. Am I saturated with the responsibility, so that sometimes (maybe all the time?) I feel that's all there is left to life?

8. *Who* am I? And *where* am I, in relation to other people? What are my interests?

9. What do I think of *myself*?

10. What could I do with my own life (something I'm not doing now) if I no longer had this responsibility?

11. What would I expect my children or other family members to do for me if I could not manage my own life?

12. What counsel might I offer to another person who takes on the care of an elderly person who is disabled?

It would require some time to find all the answers. In the meantime, I tried to put my life into perspective by writing down my priorities:

1. I must survive, and have that right.

2. Sometimes I need a few hours away from the burden, to recapture the strength I have lost.

3. I am not indispensable; sometimes someone else must act in my place.

4. Guilt trips should be brought to an end; they accomplish nothing. They are not an emblem of loyalty to a loved one whom I have wronged.

5. I agree with a friend who said, "No one else can tell me how I should feel about a given experience; because of my own personal make-up, it's natural for me to respond to life's experiences in a way all my own."

6. Patience with myself is imperative, for through this the healing of my spirit will come.

I began to consider some solutions:

1. Develop a piece of my life, so that I have a feeling of accomplishment *now* . . . so that I will have something of value to turn to *later*, when this responsibility comes to an end.

2. Choose a challenge and a goal to make life exciting.

3. Expose my life to *new* experiences that may lead to a fuller life.

4. Find a creative friend who has been through a stressful experience and gather some ideas of how he or she handled it.

5. Share some of my own creative thoughts with a friend.

6. Along the way, consult available counseling services in the community, such as churches, mental health agencies, and support groups for professional guidelines.

7. Cultivate the joy of the written word. Read and read and read; especially books and articles on personal growth.

8. Enjoy the good things that surround me; absorb them until they become as much a part of me as a leg or an arm.

9. Learn to be solitary some of the time.

10. Be lazy sometimes to relieve my tensions.

11. Work like crazy other times so I'll need to be lazy again.

12. By all means, work on a good sense of humor! Share it. Then cleanse my soul with hearty laughter.

Chapter Twenty

For years I have been a believer in "cues," or "signals," as a friend calls them. Or "divine guidance." Or "being in the right place at the right time." Or a sensitivity to "road signs" that point in the right direction.

I had reached another crossroads. I awoke in The Haven with a sense of solitude, trying to put the problem into perspective. Watching the falling of yellow birch leaves framed in the bedroom window, like bits of gold lace dripping from God's fingertips, I longed to hear a voice telling me exactly what to do.

The "voice" came from Terry Brown. "Just let it roll," he said. "These things have a way of falling into place."

Maybe so. But John had phoned to say that a substitute aide had missed a day's work (on Friday, of all days!) and the day before had left only a glass of water—no tomato juice, no milk, no orange juice. John promised to prepare a sandwich, a glass of milk, and a thermos of soup.

"Wait!" I kept telling myself. "Wait here! Winter is ahead. I need to store some of the forest and the beach and the sunsets in my heart, to prepare for who-knows-what." At least, it would do no harm to wait until the next day when John would call back after contacting the Visiting Nurses headquarters.

Promptly at nine the next morning, John phoned to say the

117

aides would be on hand definitely, five days a week. Dad had eaten a sandwich, which meant he had been out of bed.

Mrs. Emmons called again to say she had talked to Dad and, without mentioning nursing home, had suggested that he move to a place that housed other men. Dad had even agreed that he might feel less isolated.

"I'm letting the agencies handle everything," I reported to Terry.

Terry said, "Good! They know how."

I tried to steady my voice. "You've no idea how hard it is to let others take charge. I've done it so long by myself."

"It's a new way of life for you," Terry said sympathetically, adding a statement that was one of the most significant of any I had heard: "Too often people in this situation expect perfection. There is no solution that is perfect. There are choices to be made, none of them pleasant. That's reality!"

What clearer "signals" could I expect? First, assurance that the aides would come regularly. Second, the social service agency's effort to place Dad. Third, Terry's friendly, expert counsel.

Even so, my thoughts began to shilly-shally back and forth, uncontrollably, disconcertingly. Should I change my mind and agree to become a guardian? I had been told that a guardianship would give me the authority to force Dad bodily to enter a home. But I shrank from the thought of having my father shackled by the police, as one lawyer had suggested, or from leading Dad to suppose I was taking him to a restaurant, then walking him into a home. I could never lie to him, then face him later on. If someone else became guardian, would he meet my father's needs? Would a guardian insist on forced feeding, or on other life-sustaining measures when no quality of life remained?

I began to assess Mrs. Emmons's insistence that my father needed care; that he was not safe at home alone. What was the meaning of the words *care* and *safety* in the context of the life of one who was ninety-four years of age, blind, deaf, and with no desire to live? In the beginning, the doctor had urged, "Keep him at home as long as you can." At home, Dad could hang on to his last remaining freedoms, the choice of eating or going without food, of remaining in bed or getting up—while waiting for life to end.

A rainstorm pelted the roof of the cottage. I could not explain the sudden lifting of my depression, or the feeling that a new day had dawned, bearing hope. I wondered if it was raining at home. For some strange reason, I thought of Dad's umbrella standing in the closet and determined to discard it soon, along with the trauma it symbolized.

The leaves on the ground surrounding the cottage were blood red. There was no "lace" framed in my bedroom window, for the branches of the beech tree were stripped bare. The time had come to leave The Haven alone with its memories and its dreams of better days ahead.

Chapter Twenty-one

I awoke to a dismal November Sunday with an uneasy sensation. Something was wrong. Then I remembered! On Friday a Visiting Nurse supervisor had phoned, claiming that Dad had struck and injured an aide. The service was withdrawing its assistance. I tried not to reveal that I was shaken by the news. I reminded myself that I could manage, as I had before the aides came; but forced by the phone call to face reality, I had to admit that the situation was getting out of hand.

I opened the drapes to look for a light in my father's bedroom. The window across the way was dark with no sign of life. Probably Dad was huddled in bed—not dead, but not really alive, with no desire to care for himself or to be cared for, with no wish to go on living, but unable to die.

Yesterday I had wept in John's arms. "I need you. Oh, how I need you!"

"You have me," John said.

The cancer that had emaciated his body and sallowed his complexion made me wonder how long I would have him. But the determination in his eyes and the set of his chin supported his promise, "No way am I willing to let the Old Man outlive me. You still have me. Don't you forget it!"

All along the tedious road, I had had John. Whenever we

121

took Dad out to dinner John helped him patiently in and out of the restaurant, and took him out to eat when I was at The Haven; whenever I spouted off about Dad locking me out of the house or about his refusal to bathe; whenever I had had to make decisions without support from my brother. Even when John found he had cancer, he had encouraged me to put Dad's needs ahead of his.

Again and again, I had fretted, "Dad shouldn't have become your problem—he's not your father. You should be able to enjoy your retirement."

"But you need someone," John said.

After losing the aide service, I said, "There'll be no death with dignity for my father. He's seen to that: first by picketing; then by screaming at our door; by summoning the police again and again; now, to top it off, by striking an aide. You can be certain everyone at Visiting Nurses is chewing on that."

John nodded. "Even though he can't help some of his actions, the truth is, he's made a spectacle of himself. Considering all you've had to cope with, I can't understand why your brother doesn't write or phone you . . . doesn't do something to show you he cares."

"I don't think he does care," I said. There was no healing of the feeling that Frank was letting John do all the supporting. Too many dreams had died: the dream that people would remember my father's contribution to the community; the dream that Frank and Dad and I would remain a family; the dream that I could provide happiness for my father to the end. My thoughts turned then from lost dreams to the practical. I said, "I'll go next door to fix a thermos of coffee before church."

The other house was permeated with an atmosphere of emptiness, with no sound except the knocking of the radiators. By habit, I checked to see if the telephone receiver was in place; opened the refrigerator and found the sandwich, prepared yesterday, untouched in its wrapper; the bottle of milk full. On the table, Dad's favorite cookies waited in a bowl.

Commonplace sounds began to add to the loneliness: the

slamming of the refrigerator door, the hiss of steam from the teakettle, the slurp of water poured into the thermos. Long ago, I had given up listening for visitors at the door (so why have the bell repaired?). Long ago, my father's friends had stopped phoning. (Most calls turned out to be the wrong number.) Only the minister made an attempt to come, and when Dad refused to answer the door, he left his card. (No one thought of calling me to ask to see Dad.)

Had people stopped contacting my father because he kept himself locked in? (Or was this an excuse, not a reason?) Did they dread his emotional outbursts? (Or were they avoiding a reminder that someday they, too, might be disabled?) Had people forgotten my father's contribution to the community? Had those he called his friends in the Breakfast Club clasped peace of mind to their bosoms while one of their members was lonely and isolated?

In the October 25, 1979 issue of the *Wall Street Journal*, James Hyatt writes:

> "It doesn't mean a lot to live into your 70s if you don't feel good," says Dr. Robert N. Butler, director of the National Institute on Aging. At the Senate Special Committee on Aging, staff director Bentley Lipscomb agrees. "We've been adding a lot of years to people's lives, but we haven't, in some cases, been adding a lot of life to people's years."

Why couldn't life come to an end with applause? With words of praise? With glorious fanfare!

Isolation tagged at my heels as I walked to church. Loneliness followed me into the shelter of people who meant to be kind. The loneliness blocked my prayers, after the service built an invisible barricade between me and those who had stopped asking, "How's your father?" Perhaps I need not worry about people remembering Dad's outlandish behavior. Very likely they didn't care enough to remember! After church, I expected to find Dad in the kitchen, bending over his sandwich; but the food remained untouched, and the thermos was still full.

In moments of despair, Dad had begged, "Don't bring me any food. Just let me die."

And I, in my own desperation had cried out, "I can't take on that responsibility. You've no right to ask it of me."

Now he was assuming the responsibility himself. Now the will to die was taking over, as he stayed in bed refusing sustenance.

A bumping sound interrupted my thoughts. Perhaps Dad had decided to get up. I opened is bedroom door quietly, thinking, "I can't bear to have him hear me and hide under the covers."

The bed was empty, the covers thrown aside. A blanket dragged on the floor. Beside it, my father grasped the side of the bed, trying to pull himself up.

His dead weight was beyond my strength. As I dialed the police department, I tried to block out his protests, "Please don't call anyone. Just let me try. Please!" The young officer who came managed to lift Dad onto the bed, and promised to return if needed.

After other falls, Dad had recovered his equilibrium. This time, as he started for the bathroom, leaning on my arm, he began to lose his balance. Without enough strength to support him, I had to lower him slowly, gently to the floor.

Searching for the ambulance number on the emergency list was like a dream, rehearsed again and again. The screech of the ambulance siren was like a nightmare, announcing the unavoidable turning point—no longer could I or anyone else care for Dad at home. The siren shattered my father's isolation, summoned neighbors to their porches, curious about the Old Man . . . death without dignity. No dignity at all.

I faced the ambulance driver. "Did you have to make such a clamor?"

He shrugged and said someone had told him Dad had had a heart attack.

As the attendant and the returning policeman lifted my father onto a stretcher, tucked the blanket around him, and tried to quiet his fears, I became aware of his total helplessness as I watched him lose his last freedom—the freedom to call all the shots.

In the hospital emergency room, the doctor and a nurse struggled to remove Dad's pajamas. "There's still some fight in him," I said. "Let me help. I'm an old hand at this."

Other times I had struggled alone. As I unclenched Dad's fists and removed his pajama top, I was relieved that yesterday I had managed to change him into clean pajamas, and wished now I had shampooed his hair.

"He may have had a heart attack," the doctor said. "He should stay overnight for observation. Why don't you go home and rest? We'll call when you're needed."

Dad's front door was closed but unlocked, the house empty and soundless; the bedclothes and his cane still on the floor, and the room heavy with stale air.

I said aloud, "He'll never come back."

The phone interrupted my thoughts. The doctor was calling to say my father was resting comfortably, and that X-rays ought to be taken the next day. "If an emergency arises during the night," he asked, "shall we take life sustaining measures?"

I gasped. Even now I must make a decision for another adult—a life and death decision. I said, "I don't feel you should extend his life, but please call my brother and consult him."

Despite the rift that separated us, long ago I had decided on another guideline: I would keep Frank informed of emergencies. I dialed his number. Betty answered and promised to give Frank the message when he returned. I waited for him to call, but he never did.

The next day, a nurse said Frank had phoned the doctor to inquire about Dad's condition. I was glad, and reassured myself that later Frank would contact me.

Dad's voice filled the hospital corridor. "Will someone please come? It's an emergency." A nurse reported that he had fought off four of the staff who held him down for an X-ray.

At Dad's bedside, a young doctor said, "I hear you ate a good dinner, Mr. Yale."

"What did you have, Dad?" I asked.

He had forgotten, but kept talking about leaving "this place."

The doctor followed me into the hall, listened patiently as I described my father's problems and how I had tried to cope, and let me release some of my feelings of guilt. Embarrassed suddenly, I stopped, exclaiming, "Oh, forgive me, I'm not your patient."

The doctor was youthful and compassionate. He said whimsically, "Just wait till you get my bill," then soberly he said, "You've done the right thing to keep him at home. You gave him good care."

I shook my head, partly from fatigue and bewilderment, partly from a sense of guilt that, in recent months, I had not provided care that was good enough.

I wept at home later, when John said Frank had not called. As the days passed, I learned not to expect to hear my brother's voice whenever I answered the phone. I hungered for him to contact me at least once. I needed to feel we were still a family. I felt alone.

Again at the hospital, I told a nurse, "My father will never make it to a nursing home. He's going down hill."

"You might be surprised," she said. "He has a strong constitution."

But I had learned to read the signs, to sense changes, to interpret the future because I had been close to the past.

Six days after Dad had been admitted, a sense of urgency made me hasten to the hospital. He was strapped into a wheel chair, slumped over, his untouched dinner on a tray in front of him.

"I'll try to feed him," I told a nurse. "Come on, Dad, eat this sherbet. It should slide down easily."

I could not be sure whether his lips moved, but the sherbet rolled down his chin.

I rang the nurses station. "He's not responding. I am sure he's worse."

A male aide helped lift Dad into bed. The nurse checked his blood pressure and said it was low, then covered him with another blanket.

The sound of my father's labored breathing filled the room, as I held his cold hand and watched. Numbness wrapped us both, as five years of his loneliness and mine began to slip into the past. Five years of being his parent. Five years of seeing him lose his freedoms, one by one. Five years of watching him die in incredible isolation. I wanted to cry, but all my tears had been shed long ago.

I began to walk aimlessly about the room, opened the bedside table drawer and removed an envelope addressed to Dad. Realizing his breathing had become less labored, I slipped the envelope into my coat pocket. Suddenly, I felt as if I were coming out of a stupor. The room was empty of sound. My father's breathing had stopped.

I rang for a nurse and said, "He's gone."

After she examined him, she took me in her arms and said, "He won't suffer any longer." She helped me pack my father's clothing and his meager possessions.

As if in a trance, I made my way to the nurses' station. In a trance, I nodded to a young doctor summoned to sign the death certificate—at five o'clock, his dinner-time, after a busy schedule at the office.

The doctor asked, "Would you care to go into another room to talk?"

I followed him down the long hall to a tiny chapel where others had gone to beg God to save a loved one, or to weep after a loss, or to give thanks for renewed health.

The doctor offered me a chair, took another opposite mine, and said, "At ninety-four, you know your father had a good life."

I nodded, not wanting to reject the doctor's attempt at kindness by telling him that the last years had been anything but "good." I thought, "There have been too many lost dreams for my father . . . for me . . . and now . . . death without dignity."

The doctor looked too young to comprehend the problems of living to the age of ninety-four. He said, "I never had the care of your father, but the two doctors who attended him told me that when he was himself, he was a fine man."

We shook hands and I thanked him. My fingers fumbled with the buttons on my jacket and the wool scarf about my neck. "When he was himself, he was a fine man." The doctor's steps echoed down the corridor. Death . . . with dig . . . nity. Death . . . with . . . dig . . . nity.

My father had been dying for five years . . . without dignity. (Where was the old banter between us? "Honey Jane, you don't respect my dignity.")

I shoved my hands into my pockets, removed the friend's note and opened it. "Mr. Yale, we have not forgotten your contribution to our community. . . ."

Epilogue

After my father's death, I learned that a teacher of a seminar, called "As Parents Age," had been persuaded by her students to start a support group especially for persons who had the care of an elderly relative. I decided that the support group might help to resolve some of my own inner conflicts, for I was still psychologically bruised and suffered from a sense of guilt. Most of all, I hoped the group might offer me an opportuntity to contribute to others with problems similar to those I had faced.

Seated informally around a table, over coffee, we introduced ourselves. I wondered if the participants would feel I was an outsider when they learned I no longer had a problem like theirs. Another woman had come because, as a worker in a nursing home, she wanted to understand the problems faced by families with relatives who are disabled.

"We're glad you both cared enough to come," someone in the group volunteered. The others agreed.

"The hardest part of your responsibility is the loneliness," I said. Everyone agreed. On this common ground our sharing began.

First of all, we committed ourselves to attending on a regular basis of once every month over a six-month period. Although emergencies sometimes kept participants from coming, there was an average attendance of six—the smallness of the group making it easier to relate to each other.

No one was judgmental. Everyone listened patiently, with empathy and compassion, often shedding tears unashamedly with the person who was airing her frustrations. With this depth of understanding, nothing seemed mundane or maudlin:

"Mother wouldn't take her medicine. . . ."

"My father has to change the bed often because Mother is incontinent. . . ."

"I argued with Mother about admitting my father into a nursing home. . . ."

"Mother insists on her own way, calls all the shots. . . ."

Throughout the sharing, a supportive quality was maintained, a feeling that each person was reaching out to the other in a day-to-day struggle to survive. No longer was anyone alone.

One woman in the group described driving regularly to her mother's house, a distance away. Sometimes the daughter had to deal with her mother's confusion and her own exhaustion. Sometimes the daughter neglected the needs of her own family, especially those of a teenage daughter. A normal family life had become increasingly difficult. In fact, it seemed to have been postponed.

I asked, "Don't you think now that you've done all you can for your mother, you might consider directing more attention to your own immediate family, especially to your daughter, who really needs you? Before long, she'll be an adult and you'll lose your opportunity for closeness when she goes off on her own."

There was a momentary silence before she answered, "I'll give that serious thought."

As the meeting drew to a close, she asked a question that was both poignant and meaningful: "Does everyone here feel that I've done everything I can?"

The response was immediate. Unanimous! "Oh yes, indeed. You have."

She straightened her shoulders to make a new start, and I could visualize the days ahead, still difficult, still frustrating, still taxing physically and emotionally, still almost too much to bear. But each time she had to cope with a stressful situation, the group would be her psychological "vitamins," and recalling the members' encouragement, she would be nourished by their support and stand straight and stronger because of it.

At the end of six months, the leaders and each participant agreed that much had been gained, that support of this kind was needed.

Later, in retrospect, the leader assessed the experience:

> That was the only opportunity for many to ventilate their feelings and thoughts about their roles and responsibilities in caring for aging relatives. The warm caring and listening of others gave their feelings legitimacy. Since this is not a role shared by a great deal of people there is no social consciousness about how one should feel in this role. Mainly it is quietly assumed that women will take on this role without difficulty.
>
> It helped people in the group to make decisions which were more guilt free. One daughter took her mother out of a nursing home and placed her in Senior housing. Another put pressure on her father to admit her mother to a nursing home as he could really no longer take care of her. Still another admitted her mother to a hospital for acute care and refused to follow a social worker's "orders" to admit her mother to a nursing home. Instead, she took out guardianship and set down some house rules, utilized day care and shared "mother sitting" to relieve the burden on herself and her family. In addition to the shared "mother sitting," which continued after the group disbanded, some of the others planned to continue to meet in their own support group, and a few were determined to be advocates of the elderly, including publicizing or advocating for ways to support families of the elderly.

I can envision other similar support groups with a format that might include such professionals as a minister, a lawyer, a counselor, a doctor, a nurse, and a social worker, to provide information, counseling and guidance, to explore resources and alternatives, to find ways of release, perhaps even temporary escape from pressures arising in the experience. Because of the difficulties of securing funding, retirees with professional background might be sought to volunteer their services.

One area of need seems to be that of providing information about the names of agencies to call, for these vary with the community. In my own research, I discovered numerous names, under State or County, such as: the Department of Welfare, Social Services, Aging and Adult Services, Older Adult Services, and a more recent nonprofit organization called Citizens for Better Care.

An example of professional guidance that came my way, which would be useful to a support group, was a social worker's statement that sometimes an agency assumes the family can handle the care of an elderly parent and therefore, on the family's first contact, the agency might not send help. He recommended that in such an instance, the family should return to the agency with a doctor's written report on the parent, and should stress the limitations of the family. For example, a friend had to return to the agency to make it clear that he needed to return to his job in another state, and that his mother could not be left by herself all day. In my own experience, I learned the importance of saying to agencies, "My father needs help," not "I need help." If my father had had no relatives, the agency would have provided earlier assistance, and when my strength began to wane, assistance became imperative.

Recently, I met a woman whom I shall call Marjorie, sixty-five years old. A newspaper feature had told how she took care of her mother, then, after her mother's death, she brought her father into her own home. He was diabetic and nearly blind, and she attended to his needs lovingly and sacrificially.

After her husband's death, Marjorie was no longer able to care for her father. She placed him in one facility after another, until she found one that met his needs. Now she drives to see him, fifty miles round trip, two or three times a week. The newspaper quoted Marjorie as saying she felt guilty about placing her father in a nursing home.

"Why do you feel guilty?" I asked Marjorie.

"I don't know," she said. "I really don't."

"You realize you've done everything possible for your father," I prodded.

"Oh yes, I know that," she said. "But I still feel a sense of guilt, even though I realize I am not able to meet his needs. You see, I've always wanted the best for my father."

I recalled Terry Brown's statement that people want perfection for their parents, that there is no perfect solution—only decisions to be made, none of them pleasant.

Clearly Marjorie is rising above her feeling of guilt; she keeps active, goes bowling, has dinner with friends, makes new friends, and believes she has a future. However, it is sad that after her husband's death, she had no one to support her efforts to care for her father—not even her brother. Now, even the clergy whom she has contacted never pay her father a visit.

The situations to be faced are varied and endless. James C. Hyatt wrote in *The Wall Street Journal* of October 25, 1979:

> . . . due to advancing longevity, more "young old" children find they have to care for "old old" parents. A woman in her late 60s "might have a 92-year-old mother who is healthy and a 70-year-old husband in bad shape," says Paul Kerschner, a legislative and research official for the American Association of Retired Persons. "The pressures on that woman are incredible."

There is the man who comes home from his job to an exhausted wife who has been coping all day with his elderly mother, who is emotionally unstable. There is the woman who is torn between

134

devoting her energies to a crippled parent or to her husband and children. There is the couple in their seventies, who face limitations of their own and must make a traumatic decision—whether to care for a parent in their home, or to place the parent in a care facility. This is an incredible amount of emotional stress and physical strain for an increasing number of people! And in some instances it is not for a short time, but for years.

The plight of the elderly who are disabled is pathetic and commands our sympathy. So is the plight of the person who, day after day, gives up some or perhaps most of his or her life to assume the care of an aged relative. Is society focusing on the needs of individuals who carry this load? Or have we mistakenly assumed that those who support others so stoically can support themselves? Are we helping these supporters to maintain good mental and physical health so that they, too, may not become disabled as aged parents? Along with individual personal undergirding of our neighbors, perhaps more community support systems are an answer to a need that is increasing rapidly.

About the Author

AVIS JANE BALL, a native of Mason, Michigan, has written newspaper and radio copy for an advertising agency, edited manuscripts for her father—also a writer—prepared information for "The Hundred Neediest Cases" that appeared in the *New York Times*, authored a historical novel, and writes a "My Experience" column for a religious publication.

Encouraged by author Faith Baldwin, Ms. Ball has been inspired over the years by the framed and cherished note from the late novelist, which reads,

> "You'll make it.
> Love,
> F. B."